Home Nursing

Home Nursing

Muriel Skeet with
Jean Stroud

Stanley Paul, London

Stanley Paul & Co Ltd
3 Fitzroy Square, London W1P 6JD

An imprint of the Hutchinson Publishing Group

London Melbourne Sydney Auckland
Wellington Johannesburg Cape Town
and agencies throughout the world

First published 1975
© Muriel Skeet & Jean Stroud 1975
Drawings © Stanley Paul & Co Ltd 1975
Photographs © Euston More 1975

Printed in Great Britain by litho by The Anchor Press Ltd
and bound by Wm Brendon & Son Ltd
both of Tiptree, Essex

ISBN 0 09 122680 5 (cased)
      0 09 122681 3 (paper)

Contents

Introduction

Illness in the home

People want to be healthy and happy, but unfortunately most of us suffer from illness – or accidents – at some time of our lives. Nowadays, whenever possible, sick or injured people are cared for in their own homes. Usually this means a member of the family acts under the doctor's instructions. Sometimes a Community Nurse or Health Visitor calls to give help – either to carry out practical procedures or to give advice and guidance; but even with visits from professionals, the greater part of the home patient's day is the responsibility of his family.

The overall responsibility usually falls on the wife or mother. But, so that she may receive adequate rest or, indeed, in case she herself is the patient, it is essential for all members of the family to learn how to help when there is sickness in the home. Even children can help with fetching and carrying, preparing trays, arranging flowers, and providing company. Looking after someone who is ill should be a shared and satisfying experience for all the family – not a burden for one member of it.

Sometimes family routine may be affected and will need to be rearranged. But it should never be disrupted completely. The security afforded by routine is even more important when one parent is ill. Careful day-by-day planning in which the patient's routine is integrated with that of the children is absolutely essential. Older children often enjoy helping draw up the day's programme and should, whenever possible, be allowed to do so.

The patient's comfort

The comfort of the patient is nearly always directly related to the care he receives from nursing. And by this is meant not only his physical comfort but also his mental, emotional and spiritual peace of mind. These are particularly important when the illness is protracted, or terminal. Because of her familiarity with his attitudes, beliefs and fears, the member of the family who is mainly responsible for looking after the patient will be in a far better position to help with these aspects of a patient's well-being than a professional nurse.

If the patient confesses to any fears or anxieties which can be allayed only by a qualified person, the doctor or nurse should be told without delay. Sometimes the patient may want to talk things over with his spiritual or legal adviser and it is important that, whenever possible, he is given the opportunity to do so. The doctor and nurse looking after the patient should also be kept informed of his physical, mental and emotional conditions.

The home nurse

The person responsible for giving care should be gentle, quiet and confident in manner, speech and actions. She should possess patience, sympathy, compassion and understanding, so that she may help her charge adjust to pain, frustration, inconvenience and the limitations caused by incapacity. She should be tactful and tolerant, (but firm when necessary) resourceful and practical, cool-headed and calm, discreet, observant and reliable in carrying out instructions. In providing nursing care, punctuality is important – meals and medicines should arrive when they are expected. All meal trays, utensils and equipment should be washed and put away as soon as possible after use.

Personal hygiene is extremely important when looking after a sick person. The smell of stale perspiration or smoke is nauseating, and no patient should be subjected to this kind of unpleasantness. The hands must be well cared for. They should be washed before and after attending the patient, and before handling food. Any cut or abrasion should be covered with a waterproof dressing. Fingernails should be kept clean and short. Grooming is important. Hair should be kept tidy, and a clean, easily washable overall should be worn when attending the patient; it should be kept solely for that purpose.

Shoes must be comfortable, and should be changed at least once during the day. This will reduce fatigue. To maintain energy, a well-balanced diet and adequate rest should be taken. Exercise and plenty of fresh air are necessary.

The importance of following the doctor's (or nurse's) instructions cannot be over-emphasized: if there is any point or word in his (or her) instructions which is not understood the person giving care *must* ask for an explanation at once – a mistake made due to ignorance could be disastrous. If a mistake is made, or treatment omitted, it must be reported as soon as it is known to have occurred.

Nursing does not come easily to everyone – we are not all 'born nurses' – but it is usually helpful if you can imagine yourself in the patient's place and think of what you would like done if you were ill in bed. In this way you will be able to anticipate the patient's needs, and this is one of the attributes of a good nurse.

Note: Throughout the text of this book, the term 'Nurse' has been used to denote the person undertaking the nursing care of the patient. It should, however, be remembered that the use of the title 'Nurse' is restricted under the Nurses Act 1957, and the Nurses (Scotland) Act 1951, to State Registered Nurses, State Enrolled Nurses, and certain other categories of persons specified in the Nurses Regulations. Persons falsely claiming the title 'Nurse' render themselves liable to prosecution; a person is not guilty of an offence, however, if other persons use the word 'Nurse' in addressing or referring to him or her.

Section One
1. The sick room

Because illness is geographically restricting, the patient's immediate environment is important.

The general atmosphere in the sick room will be influenced by the people with whom he comes into contact; their attitudes should create the cheerful, pleasant, confident atmosphere essential for his mental health and well-being.

The physical conditions under which he is nursed should be planned with care.

Upstairs or downstairs?

The room chosen for the sick person should be convenient for the family as well as pleasant for the patient. Sometimes it is easier to have a sick person in a downstairs room near the kitchen, and where family life goes on around him. But if the only lavatory and bathroom in the house are upstairs, it may be more convenient, and less worrying for the patient, if he remains in an upstairs room.

Furnishing the sick room

For ease of movement around the sick room, furniture and furnishings should be kept to the minimum. Every effort must, of course, be made to make the patient feel 'at home', and some familiar pieces of furniture and favourite ornaments should be left in the room. Some of the items in the following list may well be found in any well-furnished bedroom, but it is essential that they should *all* find a place in a sick room.

1. *A comfortable bed.* Unless it is absolutely impossible, the patient should be nursed on a single bed and on a firm, comfortable mattress. The bed should be positioned so that it is possible to get round to both sides, and it is usually much more pleasant for the patient if he is able to look out of a window. If this is not possible, a looking-glass

11

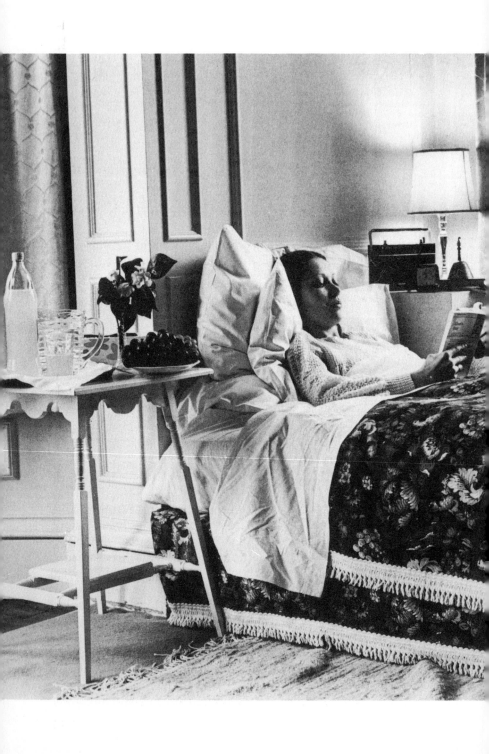

can easily be placed so that some outside activity can be watched.

('Comfort in bed' is dealt with in detail in Chapter 2.)

2. *A bedside table or locker.* This is useful for articles the patient needs from time to time and can reach himself – e.g. soft drinks, writing materials, books, a radio, a clock.

3. *A bedside light.* The patient and his nurse will find this item to be useful and necessary. It can be shaded at night if a night-light is considered desirable, and should then be placed on top of the dressing table or chest of drawers.

4. *A working surface for the doctor and nurse.*

5. *A comfortable chair* for the patient to sit in when he or she is allowed up.

6. *A chair for visitors.*

7. *Two chairs for bedmaking* (one of which may be the visitor's chair), one for bedclothes, the other for pillows and clean linen.

8. *A screen* to protect the patient from draughts and to ensure privacy when treatment is carried out.

9. *A commode* if the patient is allowed out of bed but not to the lavatory. (This can be borrowed from the Medical Loans Depot of the local Red Cross).

10. *Space* for storing equipment, clean dressings, etc.

11. A *cupboard*, which can be locked, for medicines, lotions, etc.

Ventilation of the sick room

It is particularly important for a sick person to have plenty of fresh air. One small window in the sick room may be left open all the time, but the larger windows should be opened for a short time only each day, depending on the weather.

If there is a draught from an open window, a screen (which can be improvised by draping a blanket or sheet over a clothes horse) should be placed around the patient to protect him.

The ideal convalescent sickroom allows for all the patient's needs to be readily within reach. Note how the patient here has easy access to soft drinks and grapes on one side, while the bedroom light, radio and bell are instantly available on the other.

Heating of the sick room

Unless the doctor or nurse issues other instructions, the temperature of the sick room should be kept at an even 16–19°C. If a fire of any kind is used, it must be protected at all times by a fire guard.

Used equipment

Immediately after use, equipment should be removed from the sick room, cleaned, and returned as required. Sometimes the doctor or nurse may ask for equipment to be sterilized. This can be carried out in the home, and the procedure is as follows.

1. *For* enamel and stainless-steel bowls, receivers, dishes, instruments, rubber tubing or catheters:
   (a) Completely immerse in boiling water
   (b) Bring the water to the boil again
   (c) Boil for at least five minutes
2. *For* glassware, crockery, glass and metal syringes (separate the parts and wrap in material):
   (a) Completely immerse in cold water
   (b) Bring the water to the boil
   (c) Boil for at least five minutes

Disposable equipment

Nowadays much of the equipment used by doctors and nurses is sterilized by the manufacturer. One way in which this is done is to expose it to gamma radiation from nuclear reactors. The equipment is then sealed in plastic or paper coverings and remains sterile until the seal is broken. Some articles, e.g. catheters, are sealed in two plastic containers to ensure a complete non-touch technique.

Dressings and paper towels, sealed in sterile packets, are extensively used in Great Britain. Solutions are often pre-packed in foil containers; other fluids come in plastic bags.

The non-touch method for cleaning a wound.

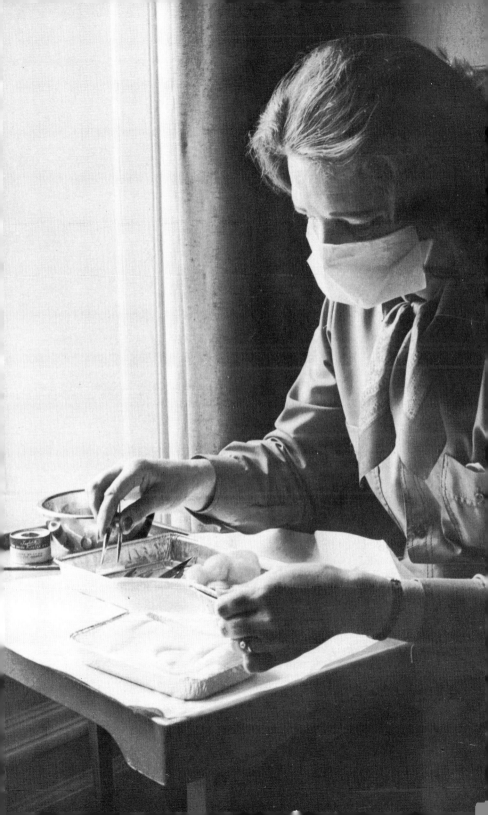

After use, this equipment should be rolled in a paper towel, and put in the dustbin.

Used dressings should be wrapped up in newspaper, and burnt. If there is no coal fire or incinerator, they should be wrapped in a double thickness of newspaper, well secured with string or Sellotape, and placed in the dustbin. The nozzle of a used syringe should be snapped off, and a needle should be bent double after use.

If it is not possible to acquire sterile dressings, the material used (gauze and wool) must be as clean as possible. Linen and cotton can be boiled, and washing and ironing destroys many bacteria.

Meal trays

Meal trays, china, glass and cutlery, should be removed from the sick room as soon as they are finished with, washed, and put away as soon as possible.

In the case of infectious diseases or infections of the mouth and throat it may be necessary to sterilize china, glass and cutlery. After thorough washing, the same procedure should be carried out as described for sterilization of used equipment (see p. 15) and any 'leftovers' must be disposed of by burning, or by wrapping in newspaper and securing in a bundle before throwing them away.

Cleaning the sick room

The general principle of cleaning without raising dust should be practised. This can be done by using a carpet sweeper, a vacuum cleaner or a damp mop. The surfaces of all furniture should be dusted with a slightly damp cloth, starting at the door and working round the room, back to the door again.

Care of flowers and fruit

Visitors do not often call empty-handed. Most bring gifts of flowers or fruit, and these require attention from the patient (if he is able) or a member of his family. If the sick person is allowed to eat fruit, a small amount should be washed and placed, together with a plate and small knife, on his bedside table. The remainder should be washed and stored in the refrigerator or larder.

The care of flowers in the bedroom of a sick person is important. The ends of the stalks should be cut and the flowers placed in water up to their necks. Then, when you have time, they can be arranged attractively in clean vases. To keep the water clean, the stems should be stripped of leaves up to water level. The water should be changed, and dead flowers removed, daily. Remember, a sick person's sense of smell is often very acute.

It is sensible to remove flowers from a sick room at night as they can be so easily knocked over in the dark. Put them in a cool place and return them after the room has been cleaned in the morning.

The look of any room is improved by flowers so, if you are preparing a room for someone who is returning home from hospital, place at least one vase of flowers on the table or chest of drawers. If it is winter and the few flowers about are too expensive, 'pad' out an arrangement with leaves, berries or sprigs of seed pods.

Potted plants also require careful attention and these usually have labels attached giving full instructions about watering, and so on. Follow these instructions closely and the maximum life span will be obtained from the plant, which will continue to give pleasure for a long time.

Do not consider time spent on these 'floral' jobs as wasted – the patient's surroundings are of prime importance and it is when one cannot get into the garden or the country-side that it is so necessary to have flowers and berries, plants and bulbs, in the house.

2. The bed, bedding and bedmaking

The position of the bed

If the patient is obviously going to be ill for some time, the bed should be conveniently positioned and of a comfortable height (26 in.) for easy nursing. There should be plenty of space around it. Light should fall on one side of the patient so that he is able to read in comfort. It should not, needless to say, be placed in a draught!

The bed should not be in such a position that it has to be moved so that nursing procedures may be carried out. Because it is now recognized that prolonged rest in bed can lead to venous thrombosis (clotting of the blood in the veins), every effort is made to get the patient out of bed as soon as possible, although some people still have to be confined to bed for a time.

The doctor's instructions regarding movement must be followed very carefully. These will indicate the position in which the patient is to be nursed, how much he is allowed to do for himself, when he is well enough to get up, and for how long. The patient should always be encouraged to move as much as he can, within the limits set by his doctor, and these movements should be increased as rapidly as the doctor permits. Prescribed exercise may be incorporated into routine nursing care. For instance, during a bed bath the patient may be encouraged to exercise his limbs as much as possible. It helps the patient if definite, attainable goals are set, thus encouraging greater effort, yet avoiding frustration and disappointment.

Rehabilitation begins at the onset of illness and every member of the family has a part to play in getting the patient back to a normal way of life. Activities of a recreational nature, within the limits prescribed by the doctor, should be encouraged, and the sick person should be given tasks which make him feel a useful member of the family – e.g. mending a favourite toy which has been broken, shelling peas, writing out a shopping list, or helping with a child's homework.

The patient's position in bed

Muscles and joints should be used correctly whether the patient is active or inactive. Attention must be paid to the patient's position at all times. He must have a firm mattress to maintain the normal curve of the spine: a sagging mattress leads to back strain and, consequently, unnecessary pain. If he is confined to bed for many hours at a time, his position should be changed frequently, thus increasing circulation and preventing pressure sores. The first consideration of any nurse, whether qualified or not, is the comfort of her patient, and there is a great deal of flexibility about the position in which he can be nursed. There are, however, five basic positions which the nurse should know and she should remember that they may all be modified to suit the individual.

1. *Recumbent position.* Lying flat on the back, with one pillow. The usual position for complete rest.

2. *Semi-recumbent position.* A comfortable position which enables the patient to see around him and eat and drink without strain. Three or four pillows support the back and the patient can move easily.

3. *Upright position.* The patient sits up in bed, with the back supported by a number of pillows or a backrest. Two pillows may be arranged to support the arms and a foot-rest helps to prevent the patient slipping down the bed. In some cases the patient may lean forward on to a bed table. This position is used when the patient has great difficulty in breathing, as in diseases of the lungs or heart.

4. *Prone position.* Lying face downwards. Pillows are arranged to support the patient. This position is used if there are lesions on the back – e.g. burns on buttocks and back.

5. *Semi-prone, recovery, or coma position.* Lying on one side with the lower leg stretched out behind, the upper leg bent in front. The shoulders are tilted so that the patient's lower arm is behind him and his upper arm is bent in front of him. The head is kept to one side. Unconscious patients

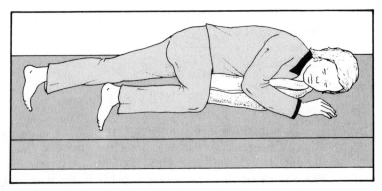

The recovery or coma position

are nursed in this position in order to prevent the tongue from falling back into the throat, and to allow fluids to drain from the mouth.

Aids to the patient's comfort

There are a number of appliances which can be used to make the patient more comfortable in bed. Some of these can be obtained from Medical Loan Depots of the Local Authority and many are provided by the Red Cross. Some can be improvised. Aids which are used in the bed must never be placed on the floor but on a chair or table to keep them clean.

Backrests

These may be fashioned either like a small deck chair or the top part of an armchair. A backrest should be placed at the head of the bed and the pillows arranged so that the patient may sit upright.

Bed-cradles

These are used under the bedclothes and serve to keep the weight of the bedclothes off the feet or legs of a patient by forming a kind of tent over them. A bed-cradle can be improvised by using a stool or a wooden box.

In addition, devices like air or sorbo rings may be used to prevent pressure on the buttocks, and wool or foam pads (see

20

Flowform Pads, p. 24) to prevent pressure on heels, elbows and the back of the head.

The following aids should be used only after you have consulted the nurse or doctor about them:

Foot-rests

A foot-rest can be made by filling a bag with dry sand and this, together with a padded board, may be used to support the patient's feet and thus stop him slipping down the bed. The bag should be covered with a sheet tucked in under the mattress. If no sandbag is available, a hard pillow may be used.

Bed blocks

Wooden blocks are sometimes placed under the legs of a bed to raise one end of it. A chair can be used instead, but it must be very firm and strong. Great care must be taken to prevent back strain when lifting a bed and at least three people are needed to raise an occupied bed.

Bed boards

Sometimes wooden boards are placed under the mattress to provide a firm surface for the patient, or level support for a broken leg immobilized by a splint or plaster.

Hot-water bottles

If a patient is given a hot-water bottle it should be a rubber one. They are much more comforting and pliable than stone or metal bottles which although good conductors of heat are more liable to cause burns.

When filling a hot-water bottle first check to see that the bottle has not perished. Place it on a flat surface and exclude all air. Then half fill it with hot (not boiling) water. Make sure that all air is excluded before you screw the stopper securely in place. Test for leakage by turning the bottle upside down. Before putting a hot-water bottle between the

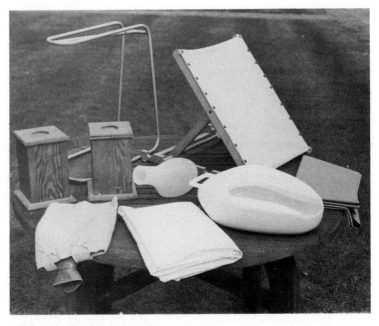

Eight simple sickroom aids:
1. Bed blocks; 2. Blanket cradle; 3. Back rest; 4. Rubber sheet; 5. Urinal; 6. Bed pan; 7. Plastic mattress cover; 8. Hot water bottle and cover.

blankets in the patient's bed, totally enclose it in a cover, making particularly sure that the metal top is covered.

Never put a hot-water bottle in the bed of a paralysed, mentally confused, or unconscious patient. They will not feel the heat, and may be burned.

Bedding
Mattresses

There are many types of mattresses on the market especially suitable for patients with long-term illnesses. These range from air and water beds to the electrically operated Ripple bed. Advice on the use of these can be sought from the patient's doctor or nurse.

Some mattresses have interior springs; others are made of foam rubber, foam plastic, Sorbo and Dunlopillo.

Mattress covers

Mattresses should be protected: disposable polythene covers are ideal as they have one open end, thus ventilating the mattress.

Plastic mattress covers are more expensive, but can be washed and dried as necessary.

Pillows

Most pillows are filled with down, feather or kapok. If necessary, plastic or polythene sheeting provides a waterproof covering under the cotton or linen pillow slip. Extra pillows are required for a patient who needs to be nursed in an upright position.

Pillows, like mattresses, can also be made of foam rubber, foam plastic, Sorbo or Dunlopillo. They are all washable.

Blankets

Woollen blankets are warm, but some patients find them heavy. Careful washing is necessary as they are prone to 'felting'. They must be protected from moth during storage. Cellular cotton or terylene blankets are lighter, can be washed frequently, and are reasonably warm. Old people with impaired circulation or painful joints may find a light *duvet* (continental quilt) preferable to the weight of blankets.

Linen

Sheets, drawsheets and pillow cases should be made of cotton and linen. Disposable paper linen is available and the quality and comfort is improving all the time.

All sheets should be wide enough, and long enough, to tuck well in on all four sides of the mattress.

Drawsheets

Drawsheets are usually made from thicker cotton than ordinary sheets, or twill, and are more absorbent.

They should be long enough to 'draw through' when the part on which the patient is lying gets hot and creased.

23

If the drawsheet becomes soiled or wet it should be changed immediately.

A drawsheet should never be patched or darned as this will cause discomfort to the patient, and may predispose to pressure sores.

Disposable paper drawsheets are available.

Disposable pads can be used if frequent changing is necessary.

Waterproof sheeting

Disposable plastic or polythene sheeting can be used under the drawsheet. Rubber sheeting is necessary if there is gross soiling and it is preferable to plastic or polythene sheeting for all children. This avoids the risk of suffocation if a child plays with a plastic or polythene sheet or crawls underneath it.

Sheepskins

For several years now, sheepskins have been used to ensure greater comfort for bedridden and paralysed patients. The patient lies on the woolly side of the sheepskin. The dense fleece provides a resilient, springy surface, and allows some circulation of air and evaporation. In addition, the wool absorbs an appreciable amount of water before it feels damp. The skins are specially prepared and can be kept hygienic by a prescribed, recommended method of washing. It is advisable to have two skins in use one at a time thus avoiding interruption of the treatment.

Specially shaped skins are used as cushions in chairs and wheelchairs, and as heel and elbow pads to prevent pressure sores in bed.

Often these can be borrowed from local Branches of the Voluntary Aid Societies.

Flowform Pads

These are made of a unique material anatomically designed to dissipate pressure, thus spreading the load-bearing area. Filterfoam allows constant air circulation and is easily washable and quick-drying. Flowform pads are available as sacral pads and heel pads. The patient should be encouraged to move rhythmically from time to time.

Covers should be changed as necessary.

J. G. Frankin & Sons, Lane End Road, High Wycombe, Bucks, can provide useful and informative literature.

Care of linen and blankets

Bed linen and blankets used by a sick person should be very carefully washed with mild soap or soapflakes, well dried and aired.

Stains can be removed as follows:

Blood: soak in cold water. Wash.

Medicine: soak in water or spirit (most medicines are soluble in one or the other).

Iodine: wash immediately in hot water and soap.

Fruit, coffee, tea: stretch material over a basin and pour hot water through.

Ink: soak in milk.

Biro: remove with methylated spirit.

If bleaching agents are used, they should be handled very carefully: too strong a solution will destroy fabric. If bleach or detergents are used, the linen must be very thoroughly washed and rinsed.

Lemon juice sometimes removes very obstinate stains.

Linen should be folded for storage. Blue tissue paper will prevent 'yellowing'.

Bedmaking

Methods of bedmaking vary with the facilities available and the condition of the patient. For instance, a very breathless patient will need to sit up. General rules only are given here.

Required bedding

Firm, comfortable mattress

Pillows. The number will vary with the patient's position in bed

2 sheets

1 drawsheet. This is a sheet about a metre or a yard wide and 1½–2 metres (5–6 feet approximately) long, which is placed over the bottom sheet for the patient to lie on.

Plastic sheeting to protect the mattress. A piece under the drawsheet is usually sufficient, but if the patient is likely to wet the bed, another piece is necessary under the bottom sheet

1 under blanket

2 top blankets (vary with the weather)

Eiderdown, if the weather is cold

Counterpane

2 chairs

Method

If possible, two people should work together to make a bed.

Cover the mattress with the under blanket and waterproof sheeting.

Place the bottom sheet in position, right side uppermost, with the centre crease down the middle of the bed.

Tuck in the sheet at the head of the bed.

Make a 'hospital corner' by:

(a) picking up the edge of the sheet about 45 cm from the head of the mattress,

(b) tucking in the sheet hanging between the head of the mattress and your hand,

(c) tucking in the side of the sheet to make an 'envelope mitre'.

Pull the sheet taut.

Tuck in the sheet at the foot of the bed.

Make a 'hospital corner'.

Pull the sheet taut from side to side.

Tuck in sides.

If waterproof drawsheet is considered necessary, place this on the bed where the patient's buttocks will rest.

Tuck it in at the sides.

Place the drawsheet over the waterproof sheeting.

Tuck in one side, then the other.

Pull the drawsheet taut and tuck in the 'slack'.

Place the pillows in position.

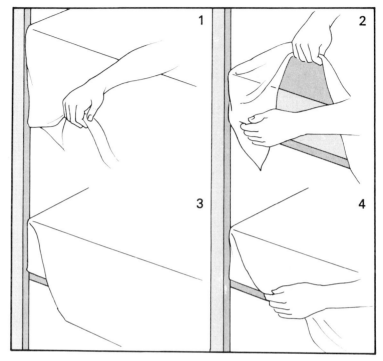

'Hospital Corners'

Place the top sheet in position, wrong side uppermost, with the centre crease down the middle of the bed.

Allow approximately 45 cm to cover the pillows.

Make a pleat in the lower end of the sheet to allow movement of the patient's feet.

Tuck in the bottom of the sheet.

Make corners.

Tuck in sides.

Place blankets in position.

Tuck in bottom of blankets.

Tuck in sides.

If a counterpane is used, tuck in the bottom only.

Turn back the top of the top sheet over the bedclothes.

To make a bed with a patient in it

If possible, two people should work together.

Tell the patient what you are going to do.

27

Warm the room, closing the windows if necessary.
Move away bedside table, etc.
Collect clean linen and place it on chair.
Collect laundry basket for soiled linen.
Place a chair at the foot of the bed.
Loosen all bedclothes.
Fold the counterpane in three, and remove.
Remove each blanket in the same way.
Remove top sheet, replacing it with a blanket.
Fold the sheet.
Place it on the chair.
If permitted, and if it is not uncomfortable for the patient, remove all pillows except one.

Roll patient away from you to one side of the bed, keeping him covered with the blanket. (Your helper will support him in that position).

Brush out crumbs, etc.

Roll up 'slack' of drawsheet to patient's back.

Pull underblanket and bottom sheet taut and tuck in.

Tuck in ends of waterproof drawsheet and cotton drawsheet leaving 'slack' at the patient's back.

Changing the undersheet without moving the patient from the bed.

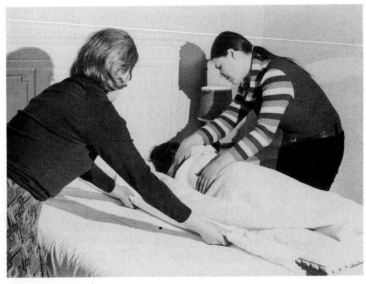

Roll patient over towards you.

Your helper deals with her side of the bed in the same way, pulling the 'slack' of the drawsheet through so that the patient has a cool, clean part to lie on.

Pull the drawsheet taut.

Roll the patient gently on to his back in the centre of the bed.

Pull the mattress up to the head of the bed (both pulling together).

Unfold the top sheet over the patient, removing the top blanket at the same time.

Place blanket on chair.

Tuck in bottom of top sheet, pleating it for approximately 45 cm at the bottom.

Make corners.

Place blankets on patient.

Tuck in blankets.

Make corners.

Replace counterpane.

Turn top of top sheet over blankets.

Replace bedside table, chairs, etc.

Remove soiled linen bin.

See that the patient is comfortable.

To change a drawsheet

Roll up the clean drawsheet.

After making the bottom of the bed, place the roll of soiled drawsheet at the patient's back.

Tuck in one end of the clean drawsheet and unroll it until it lies beside the soiled one.

Roll patient gently over both rolls to face the other side of the bed.

Your helper makes the bottom of the bed on her side, removes the soiled drawsheet, unrolls the remainder of the clean one, and tucks it in taut.

To change a bottom sheet

Roll the clean sheet lengthwise.

Proceed as for changing a drawsheet, making sure that the centre of the sheet comes to the middle of the bed.

Lifting a patient out of bed

1. Place a blanket across the seat of a chair and arrange a pillow for the patient's head. If the chair has castors, make sure they are fixed so that the chair does not move when the patient sits down.

2. Help the patient into his dressing gown.

3. Turn the bedclothes down neatly to the bottom of the bed.

4. Lift the patient's legs over the side of the bed.

5. Put on his socks and slippers.

6. Lift the patient – it takes two to do this – and carry him to the chair.

7. Lower the patient into the chair.

8. Wrap the blanket round him and see that he is comfortable and warm. A foot-stool often adds to his comfort and keeps his feet out of any draughts on the floor.

Reverse the procedure when putting the patient back to bed.

When a patient is sitting in a chair

1. See that he can reach everything he might need.

2. If he is sitting near a fire, make sure that the guard is fixed in position.

3. Do not leave him up too long.

4. Observe his colour, and if this is his first time out of bed, take his pulse to see if it has altered in any way.

5. If the patient is left alone for more than a minute or two, give him a bell to ring so that he may summon help if required.

6. Make the bed whilst the patient is up and take the opportunity, if necessary, to turn the mattress.

Moving the patient from a chair back to bed

1. Stand facing but slightly to one side of the patient.

2. Put one foot in front of his feet to stop them sliding forward.

3. Put your wrists under his armpits and bend your knees.

4. Lift him up to a standing position.

5. Make sure the patient is steady before removing your foot and allowing him to walk forward.

Turning a helpless patient in bed

If the patient is on his back and is to be turned on to his right side:
1. Stand at the right side of the bed.
2. Put the patient's right hand on the edge of the bed with the elbow slightly bent.
3. Bring his left arm across his body.
4. Turn his head to the right side.
5. Lift his left leg over the right one.
6. Lift one hand and arm over his shoulder and the other over his hips and gently roll him over.

If the patient is to remain on his side, you will need the help of another person to lift him to the centre of the bed.

Lifting a patient up the bed
When the patient is lying flat

Two people are needed, one each side of the bed.
1. Face each other across the bed, with feet apart and knees bent.
2. Clasp hands under the patient's hips and shoulders.
3. Lift together, keeping your own backs straight and letting the weight be taken by the thigh muscles.

When the patient is sitting up

Two people are needed, one each side of the bed.
1. Face the head of the bed, with feet apart and knees bent.
2. Put your shoulder into the patient's armpit.
3. The patient's arms will rest on your back.
4. Clasp hands under the patient's thighs just above his knees.
5. Lift together.

If the patient is very heavy, use your free hand to provide leverage by placing it on the mattress.

If the patient is able to help, ask him to drop his chin on to his chest, bend his knees and press his feet to the mattress as you lift.

3. General observations

If you are with a patient for a good part of the day, any observations and reports you can make can be very useful to the doctor and nurse and may influence diagnosis and treatment of the patient.

Colour

The patient may be pale or flushed. He may have pallor round the mouth; he may look blue, especially his lips. The former is present in a disease such as scarlet fever: the latter, which is due to insufficient oxygen in the blood, is called cyanosis.

Jaundice – yellowing of the skin – is present in many diseases of the liver, such as hepatitis, and also when there is infection or blockage of the gall-bladder.

Even the 'whites' of the eyes can become yellowish.

Skin

Skin is normally warm – not too moist, and not too dry. You should notice whether there is sweating and, if there is, how often it occurs – e.g. every night, every other day, etc. The skin may feel cold and clammy, or hot and dry. A rash should be noted and reported. Its type, distribution and colour is significant (see Chapter 11).

Expression

Some diseases – e.g. Parkinson's Disease – can alter the shape of a face and make it mask-like. Cortisone drugs cause the 'moon face'.

Sometimes the patient may develop a paralysis of one side of the face, or the mouth or eye may droop, e.g. after a stroke. The eyes can be sunken and dull, or bright with fever. Above all, it is important to note if your patient is

33

looking tense, worried or anxious, and to do your best (without officious probing or prying) to find out what is causing him anxiety.

Position

Abdominal pain sometimes causes the patient to draw up his knees: the depressed patient often lies or sits huddled in a corner while other conditions produce a dislike of light (photophobia) and make a person turn away from the window. All these can be diagnostic signs.

Reaction

In some serious illnesses the apathetic patient gives cause for alarm. He will take no interest in life: will not read, cannot be bothered to change position, reach for a drink, or speak to visitors. When a patient takes an interest in his surroundings, moves about and grasps any and every opportunity of being independent – he is improving! Any sign of disinterested consciousness should be reported at once.

Smell

Smell can be an important factor in diagnosis, e.g. diabetic coma. A plaster splint may hide an ulcer, and sometimes the smell of pus is the only indication of this.

Specific observations

You may be asked to keep a sharp eye open for specific happenings – e.g. after a patient has had a plaster cast put on a limb it is important to see that it does not appear to be too tight. This becomes apparent if the fingers (or toes, as the case may be) feel cold or turn blue or if difficulty is experienced in moving them. The doctor must be informed. When the plaster is dry, make sure that the edge of the plaster does not cause any discomfort or damage to the skin.

After an accident you may be asked to look out for any discharge from the patient's ears or nose. This again can be a diagnostic sign, and should be reported immediately.

It is useful for a doctor or nurse to know the temperature of the patient.

Taking the temperature by mouth

See that the patient is lying or sitting down.
Remove thermometer from antiseptic lotion.
Rinse under cold water.
Dry with gauze swab or tissue.
Shake mercury down to the bulb of the thermometer by a flick of the wrist two or three times.
Place the bulb of the thermometer under the patient's tongue.
Ask the patient to close his lips (but not his teeth) around the thermometer.
Leave the thermometer in place for two minutes.
Remove the thermometer.
Read the temperature (i.e. the point to which the mercury has risen) and record.

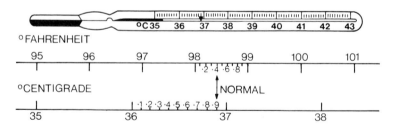

Thermometer showing Fahrenheit and Centigrade readings

Shake the mercury down to the bulb of the thermometer.
Rinse under cold water.
Dry it with gauze swab or clean tissue.
Replace in antiseptic solution.
The temperature should not be taken in the mouth if the patient is unconscious
is a baby or very young child
has an injury of the mouth or tongue, or cannot breathe through the nose
is likely to have a fit

35

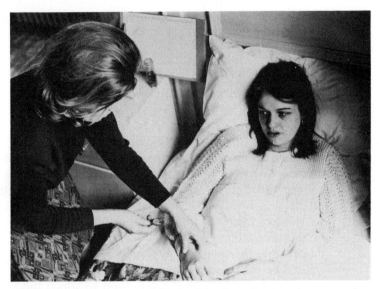

Taking the temperature and recording the pulse rate is a normal part of the home nurse's routine patient care.

is mentally confused or irresponsible
is restless and likely to break the thermometer.

Do not take the temperature of a patient who has just had a hot bath or taken a hot or iced drink, or smoked a cigarette. The clinical thermometer should be kept in a small jar of antiseptic solution when not in use.

Taking the temperature in the armpit

This method can be used for patients when the temperature cannot be taken by mouth.

See that the patient is lying or sitting down.

Wash and dry the thermometer.

Place the bulb of the thermometer in the armpit and gently fold the patient's arm across his chest so that the bulb of the thermometer is in contact with the skin all round.

Leave in place for two minutes.

Remove the thermometer.

Read the temperature and record.

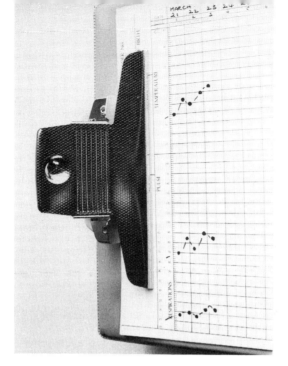

A standard chart on which regular daily temperature, pulse and respiration readings are recorded.

Shake down the mercury.
Wash and dry the thermometer.
Replace in antiseptic lotion.

Taking the temperature in the rectum

You may be asked to take the temperature of a young baby in this way.

A rectal thermometer has a short bulb the same diameter as the stem of the thermometer (a clinical thermometer has a longer and thinner bulb.)

Turn the baby gently on his side and hold him there firmly.

Grease the bulb of the thermometer with a little vaseline.

Gently insert the bulb *only* of the thermometer into the baby's anus.

Hold thermometer and baby firmly but gently and in place for two minutes, taking care that the baby does not roll on to his back.

Remove the thermometer.

Read and record the temperature.

Wash and dry the thermometer.
Replace thermometer in antiseptic lotion.

Range of temperature

The normal body temperature range is 36°–37°C. If taken in the armpit it is one degree lower and in the rectum one degree higher. A raised temperature may be due to infection (see page 123). A low temperature may be due to exposure or shock (see page 298).

To take the pulse rate

A pulse can be felt where an artery crosses a bone beneath the skin.

The easiest place to feel a pulse is just above the creases in the inner aspects of the wrist (the radial pulse).

See that the patient is either sitting or lying down.

Put the tips of your first three fingers only on the line of the artery and your thumb behind the wrist.

Hold your watch – with a second hand – in your free hand and count the pulse rate for one minute.

Record the rate.

Range of pulse rate

The average adult rate is seventy-two beats per minute but 68–74 is perfectly normal. The pulse rate is increased in fever, in fear and in exercise, as well as in some diseases.

The pulse rate of a baby is 120–140. This falls to approximately eighty beats per minute by the age of twelve years.

Taking the respiration rate

One respiration consists of breathing in and breathing out.

Count your patient's respiration rate for one minute immediately before or after counting the pulse rate whilst you are holding the wrist.

If you do this the patient will not consciously alter his

breathing rate – it is difficult not to when one is aware that it is being counted.

Range of respiration rate

The adult rate is sixteen to twenty-two times per minute.

A new-born baby breathes thirty to fifty times per minute and this gradually decreases to the adult range by the age of twelve years.

Observation of vomit

As well as noting when and how often your patient is sick, it is important to help him when he is being sick and to make him comfortable afterwards (see page 179).

If the vomit is unusual (e.g. looks like coffee grounds) keep it covered and report to the doctor or nurse.

Ensure that the patient has a clean bowl within easy reach, and remove the used one.

Disposable paper bowls are available from chemists.

Observation of sputum

Note whether the sputum is easily coughed up or whether it is difficult for the patient to expectorate.

If you think the sputum has changed colour, i.e. looks 'rusty', or has changed in composition (e.g. the appearance of pus) make sure it is reported as soon as possible.

Disposable sputum pots are available from chemists.

Stools

When responsible for the nursing care of a patient, note the quantity, consistency, colour and odour of any stools passed, and report any abnormality.

Give laxatives or purgatives only if ordered.

Urine

It is important to note colour, i.e. whether blood appears to be present, an unusual smell, or if your patient experiences any difficulty or pain when passing water.

Discharges

Any discharge from operation wounds, from the nipples, or from the vagina, should be reported. If looking after a woman with a threatened miscarriage, save all sanitary pads for inspection.

If in any doubt about a specimen, cover and save it for the family doctor to see on his next visit.

4. The patient's general toilet

Basic nursing care is doing things for the patient that he cannot do for himself. This sometimes includes washing or bathing in bed. Work firmly, steadily and evenly when washing and drying a patient – a light hand can be irritating.

Helping a patient to bath in the bathroom

If the doctor or nurse gives permission for the patient to get up and go to the bathroom, he should be supervised whenever possible. If he has to be left alone, he should have a bell within reach.

Prepare the bathroom before taking the patient to it. Make sure that it is warm. Close the windows, half fill the bath with well-mixed hot and cold water (not hotter than 37·8°C), arrange the bath mat, put clean clothing and towels on radiator or towel rail, and soap, cloths, nailbrush, talcum powder, etc., within reach. The patient should be accompanied to the lavatory first.

Giving a patient a bath in bed

Escort your patient to the lavatory or give a bedpan before bathing. When helping a patient to wash in bed, undress him, remove the top bedclothing as for making the bed, replacing the top sheet with a bath towel. Roll a second large towel underneath him. Washing all over in bed is called a bed bath or blanket bath, and is performed as follows:

1. The face, neck and ears are washed and dried.

2. The chest and arms are then washed, one arm being exposed at a time, and the patient allowed to dabble each hand in a bowl of water to rinse off the soap.

The water is then changed.

3. The lower part of the chest and abdomen and the sides

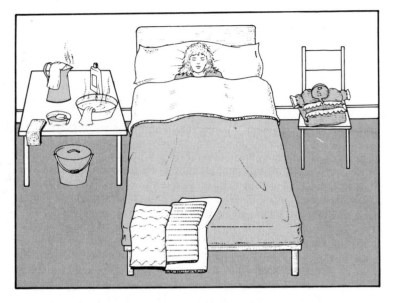

Requirements for giving a patient a bath in bed

of the body are then washed with the minimal exposure, particular attention being paid to the navel.

4. The lower limbs are exposed, washed and dried separately.

5. The back is washed after gently helping the patient on to his side. He washes the genital region himself, if possible.

When giving a patient a blanket bath special attention must be paid to washing, drying and powdering all creases in the skin: beneath the breasts, the navel, the groin, between the buttocks and the toes.

The fingernails and toenails are cut, shaped and cleaned if necessary. When cutting nails, receive the clippings into a paper tissue. Cuticles should be gently pushed back with moist swabs wrapped around orange sticks.

After attending to the mouth and hair (see pp. 43–5) the patient is helped into clean clothing and the bed is made. All articles should be cleared away, the windows opened, and the patient left to rest with a hot drink if desired.

Care of the mouth

If the patient is able to clean his teeth himself he should be given a towel, a toothmug of warm water, a bowl, toothbrush and toothpaste or tooth powder. Warm water and a cleaning powder should be used for cleaning dentures after debris has been removed with the patient's dental brush. Rinse them thoroughly before returning them. Teeth should be brushed twice daily and after meals.

For patients not able to take a normal diet, mouthwashes of glycothymolin are sometimes refreshing. A mouthwash should always be given to a patient after he has been sick.

Citrus fruit drinks or fruit sweets are useful in stimulating the flow of saliva if the patient is not allowed to drink as much as he wishes.

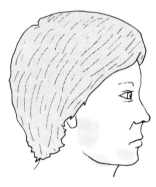

The salivary glands

Care of the mouth and teeth

The mouth must be kept clean as it connects directly or indirectly with so many other organs – the stomach, the lungs, the ears, the back of the nose, the glands in the neck and the tonsils and adenoids. Any of these organs may become infected by a dirty mouth.

If neglected, sores and crusts will form in the mouth and on the teeth, cracks will appear on the lips, the tongue will become furred and herpes may develop.

The teeth and gums require more thorough and more frequent cleaning in sickness than in health.

When nursing an unconscious or helpless patient, remove

43

sores and prevent their formation by frequent cleansing and
lubrication. When cleaning the mouth of an unconscious
patient, see that he is in the recovery position (see page 19),
or make sure that his head is in a position to prevent inhalation of cleaning materials. Cotton wool does not
provide friction for adequate cleaning and a brush should
be used whenever possible. Glycerine of borax should not
be used for the mouth of a dehydrated patient or for a
'mouth-breather'. Lip salve is preferable.

Notice the condition of the lining of your patient's
mouth, gums, teeth, tongue and the smell of his breath.

To clean the mouth of a very ill patient
Requirements

A small glass jar or tinfoil bowl containing a solution of
bicarbonate of soda – 5 ml (1 teaspoon) bicarbonate of soda
to 570 ml (1 pint) water. Beaker of mouthwash or water
(glycothymolin is usually used).

Orange sticks with ends wrapped in cotton wool (can be
made, or bought as 'cotton buds').

Paper bag for used orange sticks and swabs.

Towel (or large paper tissues).

Lip salve.

Method

Tell the patient what you are going to do.

Help him into a comfortable position.

Tuck the towel or tissue under his chin.

Dip the cotton-wool dressing of the orange sticks into
the sodium bicarbonate solution and clean teeth, gums,
inside the cheeks and the tongue, using firm gentle pressure.

Discard swabs as they become soiled.

Using the same method, rinse with the mouthwash or
water.

Apply salve to lips.

Care of false teeth

Ask patient to remove dentures and place them in plastic
mug containing cold water.

Brush the teeth under cold running water using denture brush if available and toothpaste or special powder to remove stains.

Rinse thoroughly.

Return dentures to patient in fresh cold water.

Care of the nose

Your patient's nose should also be cleaned if necessary. Young children and prostrate adults will not be able to remove encrusted dried secretions for themselves. All discharges should be removed to ensure a clear air-way. The type of discharge (e.g. blood-stained) should be noted and reported.

If a wooden applicator tipped with a cotton-wool 'bud' is used, great care must be taken: when cleaning the nose of a child remove the applicator and use the cotton-wool tip only.

A small amount of grease should be applied to the nostril edges of very ill patients to prevent the formation of crusts.

Care of the head and hair

Your patient's hair should be brushed and combed at least twice a day – and without giving pain! If the hair is badly tangled, moisten it slightly, hold the hair firmly at the roots and deal with the ends first, gently teasing until all individual hairs are freed. Only then should the hair be combed through from roots to ends.

A sick patient with long hair will probably prefer to have it plaited so that it is tidy and out of the way. Otherwise the hair should be set in the patient's normal style.

If allowed, shampoos should be frequent enough to avoid unpleasant odours and to keep the hair and scalp looking clean. If it is not possible to wash the hair, dry shampoos are available.

Sometimes it is necessary to shave a helpless male patient. This service should be undertaken with great care using, not necessarily the patient's razor, but one you are practised in using!

To shampoo the hair of a patient who is not allowed out of bed

Requirements

Waterproof or plastic sheeting to protect the bed
Bowl of hot water
Jug of water for rinsing
Bucket for used water
Shampoo
2 towels
Waterproof cape, if available
Small towel for patient's eyes
Hand drier, if available
Patient's brush and comb

Method

Explain to your patient what you are going to do
Roll back the top of the mattress
Protect the bed with the waterproof sheeting
Place the cape round the patient's shoulders
Place the bowl on the bed
Wash the hair thoroughly
Rinse well
Partly dry the hair using hairdryer or towel
Set the hair in the desired style
Dry the hair
Make the patient comfortable
Clear away the equipment

Prevention of pressure sores

Human skin can support great pressure without any ill effect, but only for short periods.

Pressure sores are the result of weight on the tissues and their formation depends on the intensity and duration of pressure. The causes can be local (external) and predisposing (internal). The latter includes serious illness, general debilitation, old age, immobility, muscle weakness and anaemia.

The former includes friction (damage to the skin), shearing (tearing of the smallest blood vessels), and pressure from an unyielding surface (i.e. bed) against a bony area of the body (head, shoulders, heels, spine, hips, sacrum, elbows and so on). Maceration of the skin from prolonged contact with moisture (sweat, urine or faeces) is another contributory factor.

It is important therefore to:

1. Prevent sustained pressure in one area.

It is vital to re-position your patient at frequent and regular intervals (see page 180). Routine treatment of bony surfaces of the body includes skin hygiene: thorough washing, massaging and drying. Sheepskins or special beds such as water beds and Ripple beds should be used where necessary (i.e. for paralysed or helpless patients).

2. Detect early the first sign of a pressure sore.

Any discoloration, redness, crack or break in the skin should be reported as soon as it is noticed, and the prescribed treatment carried out conscientiously. Once the skin is broken the lesion must be treated with aseptic precautions, using the non-touch technique. (For details of non-touch techniques see below). Barrier creams may be used for the prevention of pressure sores where there is incontinence of urine or faeces.

3. Pay attention to your patient's diet.

Loss of protein which takes place in certain illnesses, such as ulcerative colitis, or is a result of some types of trauma, such as burns, must be made up.

4. Deal with any degree of anaemia.

It is the physician's task to prescribe treatment for anaemia when diagnosed, but the first symptoms of anaemia, such as breathlessness on slight exertion or rapid wearying of the patient, may be noticed by the person who is doing the nursing. These must be reported.

Treatment of pressure sores – The non-touch technique

If sores occur – and they are manifestations of poor nursing care – they must be treated as surgical wounds and dressed, using the non-touch technique.

The patient's position should be altered to relieve pressure on the affected area. Dead tissues may need to be removed by the family doctor or nurse.

Ultra-violet light sometimes helps healing.

A watchful eye should be kept on the patient's general health and an adequate diet provided to include protein and vitamins.

The sick room should be kept clean, but do not disturb the air by sweeping and dusting immediately before a wound is dressed.

Requirements

All must be sterile. Can be bought in a pack or provided by the family doctor or the nurse
{
2 paper towels
Cotton wool swabs
Gauze dressings
Wool dressing
Small tinfoil container for lotion
3 pairs forceps
}

Antiseptic lotion – as ordered by the doctor or nurse
Paper bag for soiled dressings
Receiver for soiled forceps
Bandage or adhesive plaster to keep the dressing in place

Method

Tell the patient what you are going to do
Close the window
Wash your hands under running water
Bring the articles listed to the bedside on a tray
Turn back the bedclothes exposing the bedsore (but no more than is necessary)
Remove the bandage or adhesive dressing
Wash your hands under running water, scrubbing your nails at the same time
Dry your hands on a clean towel
Place a sterile towel across the patient between you and the wound so that the edge is resting about 5–6cm away from the wound
Using a pair of forceps, remove soiled dressing and place it in the paper bag
If the forceps are disposable, put them in the paper bag also
If they are not disposable, place them in the receiver for

dirty instruments (this should contain a disinfectant such as Dettol)

Using forceps, clean the wound by swabbing with cotton wool dipped in the prepared solution

Swab the wound from the centre outwards

Place soiled swabs in paper bag

Apply clean gauze dressing with third pair of forceps

Cover with cotton wool dressing

Bandage, or stick plaster in place, to keep dressing in position

Replace bedclothes

Make the patient comfortable

Burn soiled dressings, swabs, paper towels, etc.

Wash other equipment, and put away

Wash your hands

Giving bedpans and urinals

When a patient is dependent upon another person for this kind of assistance, he is forced into a childlike role. This can be intolerable to some people, and it is up to the person who is nursing in her 'professional mother' role to ensure that help is given and taken in the most acceptable way. Talk to any patient, or ex-patient, who has been forced to accept this kind of dependence and 'being kept waiting for a bedpan or urinal' will be high on their list of unpleasant memories. It is inexcusable on the part of anyone – professional or amateur – to cause distress by keeping a patient waiting for a bedpan or urinal.

Helping the patient with defecation (having the bowels opened), or micturition (passing urine), is perhaps the most personal and intimate activity a nurse can be called upon to do. It is essential therefore that the patient's dignity is constantly maintained, even when he is unconscious.

Two additional rules should be observed when helping a patient eliminate waste products. First, provide privacy whenever possible. Close the patient's room to absolutely everyone and arrange the physiological position conducive to normal elimination. For instance, when a patient is using a bedpan, raise the head of the bed and support his legs in the usual flexed position.

When giving a bedpan ensure that it is dry and warm: never give a wet, cold or hot bedpan. Carry it to and from the bedside covered with a cloth or paper towel. (Cover a urinal in the same way.) Take great care when sliding a bedpan under a patient's buttocks – skin can be damaged or broken by carelessness during this procedure. It takes two people to give a bedpan to a helpless patient.

Few patients are constantly confined to bed these days, so a commode or Sanichair will be needed by the patient when he is allowed up. The latter is preferable, as the patient can then be wheeled to the lavatory where the chair opening can be fitted over the lavatory pan. Even for the seriously ill, the strain of using a bedpan in the semi-recumbent position can be greater than that caused by getting out of bed on to a chair or commode. Professional agreement must, of course, always be obtained first.

When nursing a patient, note the quantity, consistency, colour and odour of any stools passed. Any abnormality must be reported. Unless otherwise indicated, prevent constipation in a bed-bound patient by ensuring an adequate intake of fluids (particularly fruit juices), fruit and vegetables. A regular bowel action can be achieved by strict attention to diet.

Failure to control the act of elimination is distressing to the patient and unpleasant for the 'nurse'. Try to prevent incontinence of urine in an elderly patient by giving a bedpan or urinal at frequent, regular intervals. On no account should the fluid intake of an incontinent patient be reduced: this only concentrates the urine and makes him liable to urinary infection. If incontinence does occur, change the bedclothes and the patient's clothing straight away. Wash the soiled skin with soap and water and dry very carefully. Use a barrier cream to form a protective waterproof covering to the skin. Special disposable incontinence pads are available. If the patient lies on one of these, change it frequently, as the skin can easily become sore, irritated, or broken. Remember that incontinence of urine or faeces is humiliating: never allow a patient to feel he is a nuisance. Dying and comatose patients are sometimes incontinent and in these cases the bladder must not get so full that it overflows. Suspect this if urine is constantly dribbling away, and report it at once to the professional nurse. The condition can be treated by emptying the bladder by catheterization.

Some local authorities have a special laundry service for the use of incontinent patients who are cared for in their own homes. Find out if your local authority is one of them.

Unconscious patients rarely have their bowels opened normally and suppositories may be ordered (see page 68).

Some waste products are eliminated by breathing and sweating. If profuse sweating occurs, the patient should be kept warm and his skin washed and dried thoroughly. It is important to remember that sweat, and indeed all body excretions, have characteristic and strong odours, and that the patient's resultant embarrassment must be minimized. Use disinfectants and deodorants whenever appropriate. Prompt removal of the excreta, all soiled linen and clothes is of prime importance. It is as well, however, to ask whether specimens of urine or faeces are required for inspection by either the doctor or nurse, or for laboratory examination. All receptacles and equipment used should be kept meticulously clean. This is especially so in the nursing of patients with some infectious diseases.

Always see that a patient is accompanied to the lavatory or given the opportunity to use a bedpan or urinal before his meals are served: mealtimes should not be interrupted because of an urgent need to use a bedpan or urinal. Similarly, try to ensure that your patient enjoys an uninterrupted rest period during the day and, of course, always make sure of a nightly routine before settling him for sleep. Some male patients feel more confident and happier if a urinal is within easy reach. Many accidents to sick, elderly people happen at night when they try to get to the lavatory by themselves. In respecting their independence, it is essential to make them aware that it will not be considered any trouble if they ring for help.

Giving a urinal to a patient

The urinal should be covered with a paper towel when it is taken to the bedside. If the patient is helpless or very ill, place it in position for him. After use, cover with the paper towel, take it to the lavatory, empty and rinse in cold water.

In an emergency a wide-necked jar may be used.

If any abnormality is noted in the urine i.e. it is blood-stained, or very dark in colour, save it for the family doctor or nurse to see on the next visit.

Giving a bedpan

Warm the bedpan by holding it under running warm water. Dry it.

Cover with a paper towel and take it to the bedside.

Close the bedroom door.

Turn back the top bedclothes.

Cover the patient's chest and shoulders with a jacket or shawl.

Help the patient to pull down his pyjamas.

Method of giving a bedpan

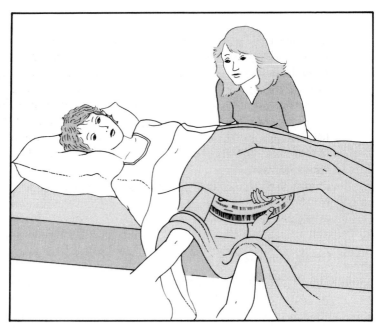

If he needs help to raise himself, place one hand under him, at the same time slipping the bedpan under him with the other hand.

If the patient is helpless or very ill, you will need help.

Give the patient toilet paper or tissues to clean himself.

If he is too ill to do this for himself you must do it for him.

Washing is sometimes necessary and this is a good opportunity to attend to the pressure area at the bottom of the back.

Cover the bedpan and remove at once.

Rearrange bedclothes and make the patient comfortable.

Give the patient a bowl of water, soap and towel so that he can wash his hands.

Note any abnormal contents before emptying the pan.

Rinse the pan with cold water, dry and store.

Wash your hands.

If the patient is a woman who is menstruating she should be given a paper towel or bag for the sanitary pad, and the opportunity of washing frequently.

Care of bedpans and urinals

Bedpans and urinals are available from the Medical Loan Depots of the Voluntary Aid Societies. Many are disposable. Urinals made of glass or stainless steel should be emptied immediately after use, rinsed, disinfected with a mild antiseptic solution and dried in an upside-down position.

A small mop (a washing-up mop is suitable) may be needed to clean a bedpan. To keep urinals, bedpans and commodes free from deposits, they should be washed in water containing washing soda.

The doctor and nurse looking after the patient should always be asked if a specimen of water or stool is to be saved for subsequent inspection. This also applies to vomit and sputum.

5. Diets and feeding

An adequate intake of food and fluids is essential to life and is as vital to the patient as an adequate intake of air.

It is impossible to generalize about a patient's diet, for much depends on the disease or lesion, the circumstances and the conditions under which nursing is undertaken.

Food and fluids taken by a patient are a vital part of his treatment. The nurse is responsible for her patient's diet and sometimes, when a patient is reluctant to eat and drink, it is necessary to persuade, coax, cajole and tempt.

A nutritionally adequate diet is a varied one. A rule-of-thumb measure is that if a diet contains at least one daily helping of meat, fish or cheese, and one portion of green vegetables, or fresh or tinned citrus fruits or tomatoes, the

Sources of   1 Carbohydrates   2 Fats   3 Vitamins   4 Protein

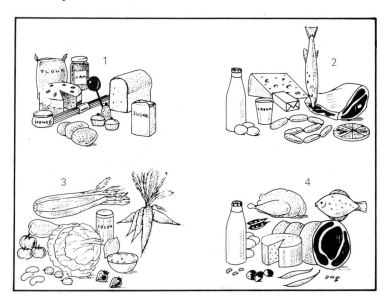

remainder may consist of foods such as bread, potatoes, butter and sugar. This is not ideal, but it is adequate – even for an adult. An important additional safeguard is milk, which is rich in most nutrients essential for healthy living. Children, particularly in early life when growth is most rapid, need a higher proportion of body-building foods than adults. They also need more vitamins, which serve a twofold purpose: they are protective, and necessary for body-building.

Although it is not possible to generalize about a patient's diet, one can generalize about the method of serving it.

Food must be served attractively and, whenever possible, the patient's likes and dislikes taken into consideration. Probably every textbook on nursing contains a similar statement, yet often one finds patients being given unsuitable, or tepid, food, portions which are too large, served on chipped or cracked plates, accompanied by bent or stained cutlery. Meal times are extremely important to a patient and a delicious meal, attractively served, will be much appreciated.

A 'normal diet' has different connotations for different people, but some attention must be paid to its composition if the recommended intakes are to be met. Foods containing protein, iron and calcium contain other nutrients. If there is a sufficiency of these items, and a daily intake of ascorbic acid (vitamin C), then the total diet is adequate. For example, a moderately active woman will require approximately 2300 calories per day. This would include 55 G of protein, 40 mg ascorbic acid, 6000 mg calcium and 12 mg of iron.

A low-caloried diet (approximately 1000 calories, with a carbohydrate content in the region of 80 G), is often prescribed for a patient who is overweight, or whose obesity has caused or aggravated a condition such as hernia, joint or back pain, coronary incompetence (a heart condition), or hypertension (high blood pressure).

A diabetic diet is ordered in the treatment of diabetes mellitus, when it is necessary to restrict the carbohydrate content. A diabetic patient who is on insulin is usually allowed more carbohydrates – approximately 180 G, evenly distributed throughout the day.

The physician must always be consulted if the patient experiences hypoglycaemic attacks (caused by a deficiency of sugar in the blood). If an attack occurs, the patient should be given two lumps of sugar or two teaspoonsful of glucose, dissolved in water, if necessary. This may be repeated within five minutes if recovery is not immediate.

A low sodium diet is given when the patient has, or is likely to develop, oedema (water retention in the body's tissues). The causes of oedema may be renal (of the kidney) or hepatic (of the liver) failure, coronary incompetence, hypertension (high blood pressure), or the administration of steroids (i.e. Cortisone).

The diet ordered usually contains approximately 0·5 G of sodium. No salt should be added to the food in either cooking or eating.

A low protein diet is sometimes given to a patient with a kidney or liver disorder. In order to provide adequate calories for energy requirements, sugar or glucose should be added to the foods. If this is not done, there will be a breakdown of body protein leading to wasting of the patient's tissue and, consequently, increased work for the kidneys.

A low potassium diet is sometimes given in conjunction with a low protein diet to patients with chronic kidney disease when excretion of potassium by the kidney is insufficient to maintain the normal physiological balance. It is impossible to lower the potassium intake by more than half, as potassium is contained in all foods except refined sugar and fats.

A combined low sodium and low potassium diet is inadequate in calories and is tasteless. Great care must be taken, therefore, in cooking and in presenting the food attractively. The calorie intake can be increased by using white sugar, unsalted butter and margarine, oil and spirits (check with the doctor to discover if these are allowed) in the cooking.

A high protein diet containing up to 130 G daily, may be given to patients with conditions of malabsorption or malnutrition. It is also used for some patients who have undergone major surgery and those who have a condition which produces a heavy loss from the body, such as ulcerative colitis.

A low fat diet is sometimes given to patients with gall-bladder or liver diseases. It is also ordered in cases of steatorrhoea, a condition in which there is failure to absorb fat. The diet should have a high carbohydrate content to compensate for the calories omitted by the restriction of fat. Protein should be of average content. Skimmed milk is necessary only if the patient feels sick or is jaundiced: it is obtainable in powder form.

Patients with peptic ulcers

It is now known that diet does not cause peptic ulcers. Small, yet frequent, meals are necessary if treatment is to be successful. Meals or snacks should be eaten every two or three hours. If it is found that the pain is worse after the consumption of fried, curried or pickled dishes, obviously these should be avoided.

Patients with ethnic or religious prohibitions

Some foods are unacceptable to patients because of ethnic customs or religious prohibitions:
Vegetarians will eat cheese, milk and eggs – but not meat or fish.
Vegans eat no animal food – and this also excludes cheese, eggs and milk.
Buddhists avoid food which has necessitated the taking of life. Their observances vary, but most Buddhists follow a vegetarian diet and eat eggs, cheese and milk.
Hindus differ in their food observancy according to their sect:
  Gujurati and *Punjabi Hindus* (and some *Sikhs*) are vegetarians. Those who do eat meat avoid beef and veal. Some sects do not allow milk, butter or cheese to be eaten.

Jews vary from the orthodox to the liberal:

The orthodox Jew does not eat shellfish, or meat which has been killed or prepared by non-Jews.

Liberal Jews will eat any food except pork, bacon, ham, sausages and lard.

Motza and Kosher margarine is usually preferred to bread and butter. Milk should never be given in a meal containing meat.

Liquid Food

All diets, whether liquid or solid, must meet the recommended intakes for principal nutrients.

For some seriously ill patients, or patients who have undergone surgery or radiotherapy to the mouth, jaw or gullet (oesophagus) liquid feeds may be the only form of diet possible.

Variety of taste is important here, and this is especially difficult to achieve when there is ulceration or soreness of the mouth or throat. Then consideration of blandness of the fluid must take priority over the desirability of variation of taste.

Unless otherwise indicated, the diet should consist basically of milk, eggs, cream, fruit juices, purées, fine cereals (such as cornflour), and sugar. Egg flips, milk shakes, porridge and milk puddings can be thinned as necessary by the addition of plain or evaporated milk. Soups and broths, to which Complan or a similar substance has been added, are also invaluable.

A liquidizer should be used, if possible, in preparing fresh fruit and vegetables, otherwise these must be strained to free them of skin, pips and tough fibres.

As a very rough guide, two pints of milk, three eggs and 2 oz of Complan, together with half a teacupful of fresh fruit purée, will supply 1700 kilocalories, 75 G of protein, and adequate minerals and vitamins for one day.

If allowed, and liked, the addition of a spoonful of brandy to eggs and milk, and a little sherry to soup, sometimes makes them more palatable.

It is important to remember that even an all fluid diet

should be attractively served. Parsley and cream can be added to soup; a slice of lemon or orange served with fruit drinks; a spot of colour in the form of a glacé cherry on milk pudding – all are important. The tray cloth and table napkin should be crisp and clean and the cups, glasses and bowls sparkling and unchipped.

Sometimes, when the patient is very weak or unable to use his arms, it is necessary for him to be given fluids. The nurse should appear to have all the time in the world (even if she hasn't!) for the unavoidable dependence on someone else, even for a drink of water, is intolerable to many patients. The table napkin should be placed under the patient's chin and, after making sure that the fluid is neither too hot nor too cold, small sips or portions should be given with adequate pauses in between. Specially angled straws are available from most chemists and these are helpful when giving fluids to a patient who has to lie flat.

Particular care should be taken not to spill any liquid, as this will add to the patient's abhorrence of his dependence on other people.

The same principles apply when feeding a patient with solid food. Again, the tray must be attractively set, the hot food hot and the cold food cold. A patient's likes and dislikes should be ascertained (i.e., how much salt he likes) and the portions given should be neither too large nor too small.

The nurse should sit beside her patient whilst he is eating. With geriatric patients, and with some psychiatric ones, it may take an hour or more to give one meal, but it is time well spent. Too often we hear of old people being served a meal, only to have it whisked away half an hour later untouched, simply because they are *unable* to feed themselves.

Physical condition (as well as disease) must always be taken into consideration. A patient with stiff arthritic fingers will not be able to shell a boiled egg or peel an orange. Many patients will need to have their food cut up for them – particularly meats. Dry, hard food will aggravate the cough of a breathless patient; a patient with a fever will not be able to eat fried food.

Remember that the gastric juices are stimulated (or not) by sight and smell – as well as by taste.

Table 1

Excerpts from 'Recommended Daily Intakes of Energy and Nutrients for the UK', from the Report on Public Health and Medical Subjects, No. 120

Age range	Occupational category	Body weight kg	Energy requirements large calories	Protein G	Ascorbic acid mg	Calcium mg	Iron mg
0–1 year		7·3	800	20	15	600	6
1–2 years		11·4	1200	30	20	500	7
3–5 years		16·5	1600	40	20	500	8
Boys							
9–12 years		31·9	2500	63	25	700	13
15–18 years		61·0	3000	75	30	600	15
Girls							
9–12 years		33·0	2300	58	25	700	13
15–18 years		56·1	2300	58	30	600	15
Men							
18–35 years	Sedentary	65	2700	68	30	500	10
	Moderately active		3000	75	30	500	10
	Very active		3600	90	30	500	10
35–65 years	Sedentary	65	2600	65	30	500	10
	Moderately active		2900	73	30	500	10
	Very active		3600	90	30	500	10
65–75 years	Assuming a	63	2350	59	30	500	10
75 years and over	sedentary life	63	2100	53	30	500	10
Women							
18–55 years	Most occupations	55	2200	55	30	500	12
	Very active		2500	63	30	500	12
55–75 years	Assuming a	53	2050	51	30	500	10
75 years and over	sedentary life	53	1900	48	30	500	10
Pregnancy 2nd and 3rd trimester			2400	60	60	1200	15
Lactation			2700	68	60	1200	15

Weight-reducing diet

Breakfast Tea or coffee with a little milk.
Either 1 egg, 1 rasher of grilled bacon, 1 slice of ham, a kipper (or piece of smoked fish), or 30 G (1 oz) cheese.
Tomatoes, mushrooms and half a grapefruit, if desired.
30 G (1 oz) bread in any form, thinly buttered.

Mid-morning, tea-time and bedtime Tea or coffee with a little milk, or Bovril, Oxo, Marmite, or lemon juice and water.

Lunch and A balanced diet of meat, offal, poultry, game,

evening meal	fish, eggs or cheese. Cooked vegetables or salad as desired. Either 30 G (1 oz) bread with butter, 1 small potato or 1 tablespoon rice. 1 portion of fruit: this may occasionally be varied by the substitution of a small helping of egg custard or junket, a plain yoghurt, or two cream crackers with cheese.

Diabetic diet

Breakfast	15 G ($\frac{1}{2}$ oz) Cornflakes. A little milk for tea or coffee, and cereal. Egg, bacon, fish or cheese. Tomatoes, mushrooms, half a grapefruit, if desired. 60 G (2 oz) bread with butter.
Mid-morning and tea-time	Tea or coffee with a little milk (1 oz), 1 plain, sweet biscuit.
Lunch	A balanced diet of meat, offal, poultry, game, fish, cheese or egg dish. Cooked vegetables, or salad, as desired. Either 90 G (3 oz) bread with butter, or 240 G (8 oz) 4 small potatoes or 6 dessertspoonfuls cooked rice. 1 portion of fruit, 1 portion ice cream, 1 plain yoghurt or 2 cream crackers and cheese. Tea or coffee with a little milk (1 oz).
Evening meal	Meat, fish, eggs or cheese. Cooked vegetables or salad. 60 G (2 oz) bread, or 180 G (6 oz) potato or 4$\frac{1}{2}$ dessertspoonfuls rice. Fruit, etc., as at lunch.
Bedtime	1 tumbler of milk (7 oz). 1 plain, sweet biscuit.

Low-sodium diet

Breakfast	Tea or coffee. Shredded or puffed wheat with milk from the day's allowance. 1 egg or a portion of fish (white).

Unsalted bread, salt-free Ryvita or Motza.
Unsalted butter or Kosher margarine.
Fruit, sugar, margarine, or honey.

Mid-morning, tea-time and bedtime — Fruit or fruit juice, tea or coffee with milk from allowance, home-made lemonade (not synthetic) or unsalted Marmite.
1 plain sweet biscuit.

Lunch and evening meal — An average helping of meat, fish or egg dish. Potatoes, rice, pasta or unsalted bread.
Fresh or frozen vegetables.
Fruit pie, fruit crumble or fritters, jam tart, pancakes, jelly. An occasional ice cream or a small milk pudding.
Sugar, jam, nuts, cream, as appropriate.

Foods for the convalescent

Unlike many of us, people recovering from an illness sometimes find it difficult to put on weight. It is important to encourage your patient to eat slowly – and to chew thoroughly. Maximum benefit from food is obtained in this way. Include plenty of vitamin D in the diet (milk is the best source). Ensure that the intake of food exceeds the output of energy. (See Appendix for calorific value of common foods).

Specimen diet for gaining weight

On waking — Large glass of fruit juice, or coffee with milk.

Breakfast — Cereal. Added nuts and raisins. Cream or 'top of the milk', or porridge with cream and sugar (if permitted).
Bacon and egg, or
Scrambled, poached, or boiled egg.
Wholemeal toast.
Butter, honey, syrup or marmalade.
Tea or coffee with milk.

Mid-morning — Glass of milk with added wheatgerm (Bemax), or coffee with milk.

	Biscuits – preferably wheatmeal or digestive, or
	Banana Whip (ripe banana beaten into a glass of milk with honey added).
Lunch (or light meal)	Cream soup. Fish or meat with salad and mayonnaise. Jacket potatoes with butter. Fruit stewed with sugar or syrup. Custard or milk pudding. Cheese and biscuits.
Tea	Sandwiches made from wholemeal bread. Tea with sugar and milk.
Dinner (or main meal of the day)	Cream soup with croûtons, grated cheese, etc., and added cream. Roast meat or poultry. Grilled or boiled fish. Potatoes – mashed with milk, cream, butter, egg, and garnished with parsley. Root vegetables (turnips, carrots) mashed with butter. Green salad with French dressing. Baked or stewed fruit. Junket, blancmange, caramel custard, milk pudding, etc. Cheese and biscuits.
On retiring	Milk drink.

Disguising milk

Milk is an essential food because it provides all nutrients (although lacking in iron).

Unfortunately many people dislike its taste and, in these cases, when it is considered an essential part of the convalescent diet, the flavour must be disguised. (It should be remembered also that cheese contains the same nutrients and $\frac{1}{4}$ lb cheese = approximately 1 pint of milk).

Soups should be diluted with milk instead of water for the convalescent. (Heat gently to avoid curdling).

Use a white sauce made from milk whenever you serve root vegetables, cauliflower, fish, cheese and egg dishes. Vary its flavour by adding tomato purée, anchovy sauce, mushroom ketchup, curry powder, chives, cheese and so on.

Serve puddings with a sauce, e.g. chocolate with a steamed pudding, fruit flavoured with sweet omelettes, etc.

Make milk shakes by adding a few drops of orange, strawberry or vanilla essence, black coffee, or peppermint flavouring, to a glass of milk. Colour with appropriate ingredient, e.g. cochineal with vanilla, green essence with peppermint. Chill in the refrigerator, top with cream, and serve with two straws.

More 'substantial' milk shakes can be made by adding eggs, brandy, honey, black treacle, wheat germ, mashed banana, etc., into either a glass of very cold milk or a glass of very gently heated milk. (The strained beaten egg should be added *after* heating the milk).

Vitamins

A well-balanced diet contains all vitamins but sometimes the convalescent patient is ordered a diet especially rich in one or more particular vitamins. The following are the most common sources:

Vitamin A	Fish-liver oil, milk, cream, egg yolk, kidney, liver, green vegetables, carrots
Vitamin B complex	Whole wheat
Vitamin B1 (*Thiamine*)	Nuts, yeast, egg yolk, liver, pork
Vitamin B2 (*Riboflavin*)	Yeast, green vegetables, milk, liver and kidneys, fish roes
Nicotinic acid	Liver, yeast, milk, cheese, eggs, cereals
Vitamin B6 (*Pyridoxine*)	Egg yolk, wheat germ, yeast, milk, peas, liver, soya flour, black treacle
Vitamin B12	Liver, milk
Vitamin C (*ascorbic acid*)	Fresh fruit (especially oranges, lemons, blackcurrants), rosehips, tomatoes, potatoes, green vegetables
Vitamin D	Fish-liver oil, butter, milk, eggs

Vitamin E	Egg yolk, milk, butter, lettuce, wheat germ, peanuts
Vitamin K	Meat, spinach, soya beans

Iron deficiency

Sometimes after a severe illness or loss of blood, a diet rich in iron is ordered for the convalescent.

Specimen diet for patients with an iron deficiency

On waking	Fruit juice or dried fruit stewed/soaked (e.g. apricots, prunes, etc.).
Breakfast	Cereal (or porridge) with brown sugar, milk or cream and wheat germ.
	Eggs with or without bacon.
	Toast with honey or black treacle.
Mid-morning	Marmite, cocoa or hot chocolate.
Lunch	Roast meat, a cheese dish, omelette – or cold beef or lamb.
	Green salad of watercress, shredded raw cabbage, etc.
	Baked, stewed or fresh fruit, wheatgerm added.
Tea-time	Brown-bread sandwiches of Marmite.
Dinner or	Vegetable or meat soup.
main meal	Liver or kidneys.
	Roast meat or grilled fish.
	Potatoes in their jackets.
	Salad with watercress cream, and tomatoes.
	Fruit – fresh, stewed or baked.
	Milk pudding, junket, or egg custard.
	Cheese and biscuits.
On retiring	Cocoa or hot chocolate.

Patients with a slight tendency to anaemia will benefit from having two eggs a day, curry once a week, and liver, heart or kidney at least twice a week. Hot milk drinks should be flavoured with cocoa or chocolate.

6. Giving medicines and drugs

Nowadays the word 'drugs' is, more often than not, associated in many people's minds with harmful substances taken for 'kicks' to which people become addicted. But in the practice of medicine, drugs are substances used to prevent disease, cure illness, and relieve symptoms.

Except in an extreme emergency no drug should be administered to a patient unless prescribed by a doctor. This applies to any drug, whether it is a poison or not, because sometimes an apparently harmless drug can produce an undesirable effect by interaction with another drug which the patient is having.

There is one simple rule to be observed when giving prescribed medicine – whether in liquid, pill, capsule or any other form. It is this: *give the right amount of the right medicine at the right time.*

Some main forms in which medicines are presented for use

1. Liquids
2. Tablets
3. Pills
4. Capsules } given by mouth
5. Lozenges
6. Pastilles
7. Powders
8. Suppositories – given by insertion into the rectum
9. Inhalants – vapours breathed in by the patient
10. Sprays
11. Ointments – given by application to skin
12. Drops – instilled into eye, ear or nose
13. Sterile suspension or solutions for injection –
   – intravenous (into a vein), intramuscular (into a muscle), hypodermic (under the skin), intradermal (into

14. Poultices

the skin), and intrathecal (into the spinal cord)
– for external use to reduce inflammation or to relieve pain

Giving drugs by mouth

1. *Liquids*

Wash your hands.

Check you have the correct bottle, and read the instructions on the label.

Shake the bottle by vigorously inverting it several times, keeping one finger over the screw top or cork. (If the medicine contains a sediment, no impacted power should adhere to the bottom of the bottle).

Remove the top (if a cork – few bottles have corks now – remove it and hold it with the little finger to prevent it becoming soiled, or lost).

Hold the bottle with the label uppermost (so that drips will not run down over the label, thus making the dosages and instructions illegible).

Hold the medicine glass at eye level and *accurately* measure out the dose prescribed.

Replace the screw top.

Check the instructions on the label once more.

Hand the dose of medicine to the patient and ensure that it is swallowed.

Offer the patient a glass of water if the medicine is unpleasant.

Wipe the bottle neck with a clean tissue and store the bottle in a cool place, out of the reach of children and preferably in a locked cupboard.

Wash and dry the medicine glass and put it away.

2. *Tablets*

Wash your hands.

Check the bottle and read the instructions on the label.

Shake out the correct number of tablets into a spoon or egg cup.

Check the instructions on the label once more.

Give the tablets and a glass of water to the patient and watch him swallow them.

Store the bottle of tablets well away from the reach of children, and in a locked cupboard.

If the patient finds the tablets too large to swallow, they should be broken into smaller pieces. If even these are too difficult for him, crush the tablets between two spoons and give the resulting powder in a spoonful of jam or honey or with a glass of water.

3. *Capsules and pills*

Do not attempt to break or cut these.
Give them in the same way as whole tablets.

4. *Lozenges/pastilles*

Give these in the same way as capsules and pills, instructing the patient to suck them and not to swallow them whole.

5. *Powders*

Wash your hands.

Mix the powder with a spoonful of jam or honey, or stir it into a glass of water until dissolved.

Give to the patient *immediately* after mixing.

Giving drugs by rectum (back passage)

To give a suppository
Requirements:
   Suppositories (remove the foil wrapping).
   Small bowl of hot water.
   Disposable glove or finger stall (obtainable at any chemist).
   Commode or bedpan.

Method

Explain to the patient what is going to happen, and see that he empties his bladder (passes urine).

Wash your hands.

Check the label for drug dosage and instructions.

Ask the patient to lie on his left side with his knees well drawn up towards his chin and with his buttocks near the side of the bed.

Tell him to breathe in and out through his mouth.

Put the glove or finger stall on.

Dip the suppository (for a second only) into the bowl of hot water.

Insert the suppository into the rectum, gently pushing it up.

If more than one is to be given, insert the second suppository in the same way.

Remove the finger stall.

Make the patient comfortable (putting a pad of cotton wool under him for reassurance if he is anxious about soiling the bed) and encourage him to retain the suppository.

Wash your hands.

If the suppository contains a drug to induce bowel action, note the stool, its colour, size and consistency.

If the suppository contains a drug to induce sleep, settle the patient for the night.

If the suppository contains a drug to relieve a symptom, i.e. pain, breathlessness or sickness, note its effect and report to the doctor on his next visit.

Giving drugs by inhalation

By this method the volatile drug is added to boiling water contained in a Nelson's inhaler or jug, and the patient is instructed to inhale the impregnated steam.

Requirements:

Nelson's inhaler or jug.

Cover for the inhaler or jug.

Flat-bottomed bowl, or tray.

Kettle of boiling water.

Bottle of drug (tincture of benzoin co. is often used in instances of upper respiratory tract infection i.e. cold or inflammation of the throat).

Measure for drug (probably an old teaspoon).

Large turkish towel.

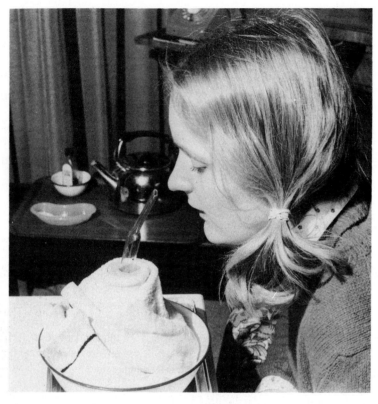

Inhalation scene. Essential aids in background.

Method

Tell the patient what has been ordered for him.

Sit him up in a comfortable position with a table in front of him.

Pour hot water into the jug or inhaler. If the latter is being used do not pour water above the level of the hole of the spout.

Pour the correct dosage of the drug (see method of pouring a liquid medicine described above) on to the surface of the water.

If a Nelson's inhaler is being used, replace the mouthpiece, making sure that it points away from the spout.

Tie on the protecting cover.

Take the inhaler in the bowl, or on the tray, to the patient's table.

Ensure that the mouthpiece points in the opposite direction from the spout.

Instruct the patient to enclose the mouthpiece with his lips, and to breathe in through his mouth and out through his nose for ten minutes.

If a jug is being used, cover the patient's head and the inhaler with the towel, making a 'tent' of steam for the

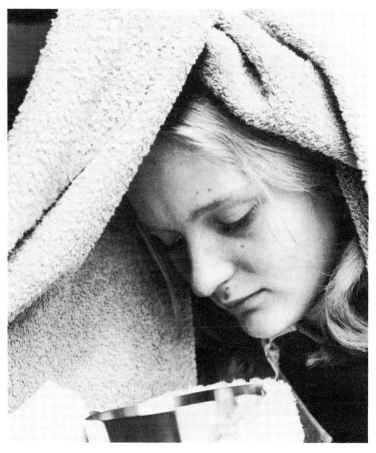

For effective inhalation the towel should completely cover the head and inhalation unit. This picture shows the correct position to be adopted immediately before the inhalation process starts and the towel is lowered.

patient. A variation on this method is to enclose the jug and the patient's nose and mouth only with a smaller towel. This method has the advantage of preventing the eyes from watering and saves a hair style from being damaged. An elderly, confused or very young patient having an inhalation should not be left unattended.

Sprays

Sprays are preparations of drugs in an aqueous (watery), alcoholic, or glycerin-containing base, and are applied to the nose or throat by means of an atomizer.

Sprays used in the treatment of asthma and similar conditions should be used with a special attachment called a nebilizer which produces a 'dry mist'.

Ointments

These are semi-solid preparations containing one or more medicaments dissolved or dispersed in a suitable base. They are applied externally (i.e. Golden Eye ointment to the eyelid).

Soft paraffin or lanolin is normally used as the base. Although some of the newer bases have a greasy appearance they are capable of emulsifying in water and can therefore be removed from the skin more easily.

Great care should be exercised to prevent contamination when using eye ointments.

Drops

Ear drops are watery solutions or suspensions of drugs (often antibiotics).

They are instilled into the ear by means of a dropper.

Eye drops are sterile, watery or oily solutions or suspensions of drugs for instillation into the eye by means of a dropper. They usually contain drugs which kill bacteria or numb or soothe the eye.

Nose drops may contain drugs which kill bacteria, numb the nose, or cause the closure of blood vessels, i.e. in cases of nose-bleeding.

To instil eye drops

Tell the patient what is going to happen.
Check by reading the instructions and dosage.
Warm the drops by standing the bottle in a small bowl of warm water. (If the drops contain an antibiotic do *not* heat them).
Wash your hands.
Draw up the drops.
Stand behind the patient and ask him to look up.
Hold the dropper horizontally with your hand resting on the patient's temple, apply slight pressure to the lower lid and insert the drops into the space so formed.
Remove your hand, and instruct the patient to close his eye. Wipe away any excess liquid.
Tell the patient to blink: this distributes the drops (and therefore the drug) over the whole surface of the eye.

To instil ear drops

Tell the patient what is going to happen.
Check the label on the bottle for drug, dosage and instructions.
Warm the drops by standing the bottle in a small bowl of warm water.
Ask the patient to lie on his side with the affected ear uppermost.
Wash your hands.
Place a small towel under the patient's ear.
Draw up the drops.
Rest the tip of the dropper on the ear opening and allow the drops to trickle into the ear.
Instruct the patient to remain in the same position for a few minutes until the drops have disappeared.

To instil nose drops

Tell the patient what is going to happen.
Check the label on the bottle for drugs, dosage and instructions.
Wash your hands.
Ask the patient to tilt his head right back.

Draw up the drops.

Insert the tip of the dropper inside one nostril and release the drops.

Repeat for the second nostril.

Instruct the patient to sniff.

Subcutaneous or hypodermic injection

This is a method by which the drug is injected just under the skin. It is employed in instances where the drug does not remain potent when administered by mouth, owing to its action being affected by digestive juices.

It is the method which has to be most often used by lay people, e.g. by diabetics who give themselves insulin.

Requirements

Sterile hypodermic syringe and needle. (Disposable syringes are widely used and are supplied in sealed plastic containers, sterilized and ready for use. Glass and metal syringes must be sterilized by boiling for five minutes and assembled with forceps).

Wool swabs (cotton-wool balls).

Antiseptic skin lotion or spirit. (Instead of cotton wool and antiseptic skin lotion, special inpregnated swabs can be bought).

Receiver (kidney dish or bowl).

Scissors.

The drug. If an ampoule (small glass container), a file will be needed to break the neck.

Method

Tell the patient what you are going to do.

Wash your hands.

Check the drug, dosage and time.

If the drug is in a rubber-capped bottle (as is insulin), swab the cap with spirit.

If the drug is in a glass ampoule, file across the neck of the ampoule, then hold in a swab whilst snapping off the end.

74

Cut off the end of the plastic container near the piston of the syringe.

Withdraw the syringe from the container, being careful not to contaminate the needle by bringing it into contact with anything.

Draw up the solution into the syringe (either from the open ampoule or by piercing the rubber cap).

Hold the syringe upright and slowly press the plunger until all air is expelled and a bubble of liquid appears at the end of the needle.

Replace the syringe and needle in the container, place in a receiver and carry to the patient.

Swab the skin of the proposed place of the injection (the outer aspect of the arm or leg are good places).

Hold the limb so that the skin is taut (i.e. stretch by pressure of the thumb and forefinger of the left hand, or grasp the tissue firmly).

Insert the needle beneath the skin, parallel to the surface.

Relax the grasp of the tissue whilst injecting the drug slowly (but not *too* slowly) and gently, by exerting steady pressure on the piston of the syringe with the thumb.

Withdraw the needle quickly and, as it leaves the skin, place a swab over the site of the injection and hold it there for a few minutes.

Care must be taken to avoid injecting fluid into a vein.

Intramuscular injection. By this method the drug is injected into a muscle. It should be used by professionals only. More rapid absorption is obtained and it is the route used for the administration of antibiotics, liver, gold preparations and hormones.

Intravenous injection. The injection of drugs into a vein is employed in order to obtain immediate effect, e.g. the administration of insulin to a patient in a diabetic coma. This method should be used only by members of the medical profession.

All disposable syringes should have their nozzle broken and all disposable needles should be bent over before being thrown away.

Poultices

Poultices are sticky paste preparations for external use, usually employed with the object of reducing inflammation or relieving pain. Kaolin Poultice BP is one of the few remaining poultices in current use.

It contains kaolin, boric acid, methyl salicylate, peppermint oil, thymol and glycerine.

It should be kept in an air-tight container.

Requirements

Tin of Kaolin Poultice BP
Saucepan of boiling water
An old knife or fork
Piece of linen the same size as the poultice needs to be
Piece of cotton wool 2½ cm larger all round than the poultice needs to be
Open-weave bandage

Method

Heat the tin of kaolin mixture in the saucepan of boiling water.

Spread the heated poultice on to the material with an old knife or fork handle.

Carry between two warm plates to the patient.

Test on your own arm to ensure it is not too hot.

Apply to the affected area.

Cover with cotton wool.

Bandage in position.

When the poultice is removed the skin should be washed and carefully dried, or wiped over with a little warmed olive oil. Particles of poultice may also be removed with olive oil swabs.

Powder the skin and cover with a thin layer of cotton wool kept in place by an open-weave bandage.

Some terms used in connection with drugs

Tolerance is said to have developed when a patient requires increased doses of a drug to obtain the effect previously obtained with smaller doses. Sleeping pills are an example.

Idiosyncracy implies a grossly abnormal reaction to a **drug** and is probably due to a genetic abnormality.

Hypersensitivity is due to an antibody – antigen reaction. e.g. a patient who is hypersensitive to penicillin must have been exposed to the antibiotic on a previous occasion without ill effect.

Cumulation. If a drug which is slowly excreted is given too frequently, a toxic level is built up. This applies to drugs such as digitalis.

It is important, therefore, that drugs should be administered at the rate at which they will be used by the body. For this reason, some drugs have to be given four times a day; others only once a day.

The date, time, dosage and route of any drug given should be recorded, together with any reaction/response/effect.

Some abbreviations used in prescriptions

Although the use of Latin in the writing of prescriptions and labels is actively discouraged, a long-established habit takes some time to lose completely.

Here are some common abbreviations which may sometimes be seen on medicine labels used in prescriptions today.

Abbreviation	Latin	English
a.c.	ante cibum	before food
a.q.	aqua	water
aq.ad.	aquam ad	water up to
aq.dest.	aqua destillata	distilled water
b.	bis	twice
b.i.d.	bis in die	twice a day
c.	cum	with
d.	die	day
ex.aq.	ex aqua	in water
garg	gargarisma	a gargle
gutt	gutta	a drop
G or gm	Gramma	a gram

Abbreviation	Latin	English
m	mane	in the morning
m et n	mane et nocte	morning and night
mist	mistura	a mixture
n	nocte	at night
p.c.	post cibum	after food
q.d. or q.i.d.	quaterdie, or quater in die	four times a day during the 24 hours
q.q.h.	quaque quarta hora	every four hours
q.s.	quantum sufficit	as much as is required
stat.	statim	immediately
t.	ter	three times
t.i.d.	ter in die	three times a day
t.d.s.	ter die sumendum	to be taken three times a day
ung	unguentum	ointment

Metric measurements and milliequivalents

Unit of weight = 1 gram.

Internationally the abbreviation for gram is recognized as 'g'. In the UK, however, to avoid possible confusion with the abbreviation for grain ('gr') 'G' is recommended as the abbreviation for gram.

1000 micrograms = 1 milligram (mg)
1000 milligrams = 1 gram (G)
1000 grams = 1 kilogram (kg)

Unit of volume = 1 millilitre
1000 millilitres (ml) = 1 litre (l)

Unit of length = 1 metre (used for length and width of bandages)
100 centimetres (cm) = 1 metre

Metric and imperial equivalents (Approximate)

1 milligram = 1/60 grain (gr)
60 milligrams = 1 grain
1 gram = 15 grains
30 grams = 1 ounce (oz)

1 kilogram (kg)	= 2¼ pounds (lb)
6·5 kilograms	= 1 stone

1 millilitre	= 15 minims (m)
30 millilitres	= 1 fluid ounce (fl oz)
600 millilitres	= 1 pint (pt)
1 litre (l)	= 35 fluid ounces

1 millimetre (mm)	= 0·0394 inch (1/25 approx)
1 centimetre (cm)	= 0·394 inch (2/5 approx)
1 metre (100 cm)	= 39·37 inches (1 yard 3¼ inches approx)

1 inch	= 25·4 mm
1 foot	= 30·5 cm
1 yard	= 91·5 cm

Section Two

7. Care of the young baby

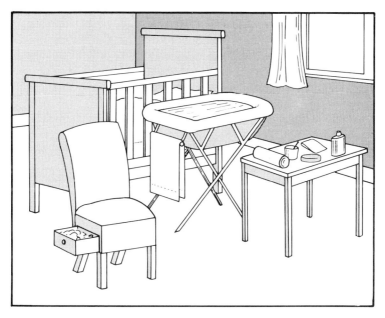

Furniture for a baby

Although parenthood is perhaps the most important 'career' of all, many parents embark upon it with little or no training or preparation.

Instinct usually provides the urge to care for and protect offspring; it does not necessarily provide adequate knowledge of how to do it.

The expectant mother can receive instruction in mother-craft from the family doctor, or from the doctor, midwife or health visitor at the ante-natal clinic. After the birth of the baby, regular visits from the midwife and health visitor, and visits to the clinic or health centre, provide an opportunity for questions to be asked and advice to be given.

The father has an important part to play in the early stages of his child's life, not only in seeing that the child's

81

mother keeps fit by continuing her ante-natal routine of taking plenty of fresh air, exercise and rest, and keeping to a well-balanced diet, but also in helping her with feeding and changing the infant.

A shopping expedition to buy baby's layette is a most enjoyable experience for any parent, but it can be confusing to be confronted by the wide range available in today's shops and stores. It is wise to do this shopping early in pregnancy when it is less tiring; then you can sit with your feet up, knitting, during the last few weeks! (Not, of course, omitting the usual daily walks and exercises).

The minimum number of garments should be bought because the baby will doubtless be given a number of clothes when it is born. Baby clothes should be warm, soft, light in weight, porous, non-inflammable, easy to wash, non-irritating to delicate skins, and of good wearing quality. Clothes should be loose, free from constriction, easy to put on and take off, easy to wash, dry, and iron, and be simple, yet attractive, in design.

Babies grow rapidly during the first few months and this should be borne in mind when shopping.

Great care should be taken when washing woollens so that they remain soft and retain their shape. Warm water and good quality soap flakes or liquid should be used. Squeeze the article gently – never rub; rinse at least twice in clear water of the same temperature. Remove surplus water by wrapping in a dry towel, and lay the garment flat to dry (outdoors, if possible).

The minimum requirements for a baby's layette are:
3 vests
3 stretch suits
3 cardigans
3 pairs plastic pants
3 bonnets (for cold weather)
2 cellular blankets (or flannelette sheets)
2 doz turkish towelling (or disposable) nappies.

Vests

Hand-knitted vests are cheaper even when made from good quality wool, but they become felted and hard unless washed with very great care. Cross-over vests should be avoided as these tend to gape when baby becomes active, and therefore give inadequate protection from cold.

Nappies

Terry towelling nappies are absorbent, durable and comfortable. Special one-way liners such as Marathon and Everdri allow urine to pass through to the towelling nappy leaving the layer next to the skin dry.

However, this special drying action is ruined by even the smallest amount of grease, so care must be taken when using them.

Disposable nappies are quick and clean to use, and are especially convenient when travelling.

Plastic pants

Again, great care should be taken when plastic pants are used. They should be discontinued at once if the baby's buttocks become sore. Frequent washing and sterilizing is essential.

Gowns

For everyday use these have been replaced largely by stretch suits which are warm, easy to wash and dry, and require no ironing. Separate bootees are not needed.

Cardigans

These are more practical than matinée jackets as they button up the front and therefore afford better protection. They should be simple in design: 'lacy' patterns should be avoided as small fingers can so easily get caught up in the holes. Flat buttons are the best: check that they are sewn on very, very securely.

Bonnets

Again, these should be simple, knitted in light-weight wool, and used only in cold weather.

Shawls

Shawls have been mostly replaced by cellular blankets which are both light and warm, and easy to wash and dry, but light wool shawls are useful especially at feeding times.

Bibs and feeders

Bibs are made from many materials these days. Plastic bibs are dangerous and can cause suffocation unless safely secured around the waist, so always tie them down.

Turkish towelling is absorbent and easy to wash. Disposable bibs have an obvious advantage.

Cold and the young baby

The importance of clothes and clothing for the new born baby has been emphasized, because babies are liable to become chilled during the first few weeks of life.

Most people know that premature babies require careful protection from chilling, but it is not so widely known that if full-term babies are not kept sufficiently warm and their body temperature falls below a certain point, then serious harm may result from what is now called 'cold injury'. This can be serious and death may result.

Advance preparations should be made so that chilling is avoided.

Reasons for vulnerability to cold

New-born babies are more susceptible to chilling than older children and adults because:

1. They have an unusually large surface in relation to weight from which to lose heat.

2. At birth the body surface is wet: when drying, evaporation takes place and loss of heat occurs.

3. They have not the ability to shiver.

4. Their metabolism and heat production does not begin until they are a few days old.

5. They are inactive and drowsy. When they begin to feed, cry, and move their limbs, their heat production increases.

Symptoms to watch out for

The onset of 'cold injury' is insidious and can be missed. Some of the most important indications are the appearance of the cheeks, hands and feet. In cases of extreme chilling, these will be lobster red and this gives the baby a misleadingly 'healthy' look.

When the temperature falls to a dangerous level (32°C or lower) the baby:

becomes quiet and difficult to rouse

looks 'placid'

is difficult to feed

is cold to touch (this is often first noticed when the baby is brought into contact with the breast for feeding)

develops 'puffiness' of hands, feet and, sometimes, eyelids. Babies are most at risk for the first three months of their lives and in Great Britain, at any rate, during winter-time, from November – March.

If the baby is delivered at home, the midwife will see that the room is warm. When the baby arrives, the temperature should be maintained and, in and around the cot, should be not less than 21°C, day and night. It is advisable to keep a wall thermometer in the baby's room so that regular checks can be made. In cold weather also check the baby's body temperature. This can best be done when handling him for feeding, changing and loving, by feeling his face, hands and feet. If they feel cold, the doctor or midwife must be told at once, so that the baby's temperature can be checked. Never warm a baby by taking him into bed with you if you are alone. Do this only when the midwife or some other person is in the room. This is to guard against your overlaying the baby if you should happen to drop off to sleep.

Heating applicances

A hot-water bottle should be used for warming the cot only. It must always be removed before putting the baby into the cot. If it is left in, there is a risk that the baby may be burned or scalded.

If a coal fire is used, it must be kept alight during the night when the temperature drops.

Electric fires tend to dry the air. Paraffin heaters are a fire hazard.

Because of the frequent fall in gas pressure at night, it is imperative to see that gas fires are not turned down too low.

All fires must be guarded: this is especially important if there are other children in the house.

Diarrhoea and vomiting (infantile gastro-enteritis)

This is a condition in which babies are sick frequently, and pass very loose motions. It may be caused by many different organisms, and is infectious.

In most cases, the attack is mild: but sometimes attacks can be severe – even fatal. Dehydration – lack of water – is the symptom which must be prevented. It can be recognized by signs of restlessness, dry tongue and throat, loss of weight and a 'pinched' appearance of the face.

At the onset of loose stools and sickness, the family doctor or health visitor should be informed immediately. No food, but plenty of fluids (not milk) should be given (see Chapter 5).

To prevent attacks great care must be taken when making up bottle feeds. Hands should be washed before and after; all utensils should be kept scrupulously clean and totally immersed in Milton (or similar solution) when not in use. Flies are a great source of danger and must be kept away from bottles and teats.

Feeding a baby

Most mothers are anxious to do what is best for baby and the natural food for a baby is its own mother's milk. There are, however, mothers who for very good reasons cannot feed their babies and whilst everything should be done to encourage breast feeding, a mother has not failed if this is not achieved.

Breast feeding may not be possible for a variety of reasons. The mother may be ill, the milk supply may be inadequate, the breasts may be ill-developed or damaged. Other mothers may not wish to breast feed for social, economical, or emotional reasons. The wishes of the mother are as important as the needs of the baby. Satisfactory feeding depends on a contented baby and a happy mother.

On the whole, breast feeding is easier than bottle feeding. The milk does not need to be sterilized or warmed. It does not have to be specially stored, nor prepared before use. It is sometimes said that there is a closer emotional relationship between the breast-fed baby and its mother than there is between the bottle-fed baby and its mother.

There is some evidence that breast-fed babies acquire additional immunity to certain diseases but this has not been proved. Breast feeding does not permanently affect the shape of the breasts.

Providing the mother has a reasonable diet, the baby will obtain all the nourishment necessary. The only supplements needed by some breast-fed babies in the United Kingdom are certain vitamins and, sometimes, iron.

There is little difference between the cost of breast feeding and bottle feeding in this country because of the welfare state, with allowances available to mothers and children.

Bottle-fed babies thrive as well as breast-fed babies in so far as weight gain and other measurements are concerned. Indeed, some experts state that bottle-fed babies in this country tend to be too fat.

Preparation of the baby for feeding

After the mother has washed her hands, breasts and nipples the baby should be picked up and his napkin changed, so that he is comfortable. He should be loosely wrapped in a shawl or light blanket.

A comfortable position for mother and baby is essential. Most mothers find a low chair more comfortable than one of ordinary height. A small pillow or cushion may be placed under the mother's elbow supporting the baby's head. Some babies feel for the nipple; others wait for mother to put the nipple into his mouth. This is best done by supporting the breast with fingers below and the thumb on top. The baby will squeeze with his lips, if necessary; no squeezing is needed by the mother. Care should be taken to see that the baby's nose is not covered by the mother's breast, otherwise he will need to breathe through his mouth.

Breast milk is very different from cow's milk: it looks like water.

Some mothers, seeing this watery fluid, feel that it cannot be good enough to provide nutrition: this is not so, of course, but if there is any doubt or fear, the doctor or health visitor will advise.

Timing of feeds

Some doctors recommend fixed feeding times but the majority of mothers prefer the relative freedom of demand feeding. Babies on a self-demand programme soon acquire a routine of their own, and often feeding times will be found to occur at or about the same time each day.

Some mothers feel it is wrong to give the baby a feed during the night and, indeed, very often babies will sleep from ten or so at night until 6 a.m. But it is not wrong to feed a baby during the night. If he cries, decide whether it is due to hunger or not. If it is, a little water may be offered, but it is probably better to feed him straight away.

The most important aim is to find a regime which fits into daily commitments so that the husband and other children do not feel neglected, and mother does not get overtired and harassed!

The amount a baby should take and how long it should spend at its feeds should be discussed with the health visitor or doctor. But feeding times should be regarded not only as times when the baby has food, but also times when a mother gets to know and love her child.

Wind and colic

Because their suckings always contain some air, most babies get wind.

It is usually best to pause half-way through a feed, place the baby against your shoulder and gently pat him on the back.

Make sure that his body is straight from stomach to mouth. Some mothers find it more convenient to sit the baby up on their laps and gently rub their back. Often a little food is brought up when the baby burps. This does not matter – except to the mother. Protect yourself! Some babies suffer from colic i.e. spasm of the gut. They cry, refuse to be fed and will not 'burp'. Expert advice should always be sought. Others cry during the 6–10 p.m. period. This usually stops at about thirteen weeks and consequently has been named 'the three-month colic'. What causes it is not known. Again, if this is worrying, the health visitor or doctor should be consulted.

Supplementary and complementary feedings

Some mothers who wish to breast feed find their supply of milk is inadequate. The more worried and anxious the mother, the longer it will take to produce enough milk to satisfy baby. Proper preparation of the breasts before feeding times is important. Relaxation is vital.

If, in spite of all preparations, relaxing and professional advice, supplies of milk are still inadequate, an additional feed may be suggested. If given as a bottle feed after the breast feed it is called complementary feeding. If breast feeding is occasionally replaced by bottle feeding it is called supplementary feeding.

There are many varieties of milk on the market which are suitable for baby feeds and there are a few which are not.

Cows' milk has less sugar than human milk, and it has been the practice for many years to add sugar. It could be the reason for some tooth decay. Cows' milk also contains more protein than human milk. Dried milk powder; evaporated unsweetened milk; condensed sweetened milk and modifications of these are all used.

Evaporated milk is more expensive than dried milk. Evaporated skimmed milk is not suitable for babies.

Condensed milk is used only for a very short time when a high sugar content is required. It should never be used without the advice of a doctor or health visitor.

Preparation of feeds

When preparing feeds for a baby, contamination from germs must be avoided at all costs.

The hands must be washed and all utensils sterilized.

Sterilization of bottles and teats

(1) *Requirements*

Large bowl
Glass jug
Small glass to cover teats
Plastic spoon and fork
Bottles and teats
Hypochlorite solution
Salt

(2) *Method*

(a) *Cleaning*

Immediately after use, rinse bottle and teat inside and out with cold water.
Wash in warm water, using a mild washing-up liquid.
Rinse thoroughly.
Rub salt inside and outside the teat.
Rinse thoroughly.

(b) *Sterilizing*

Immerse bottle, spoon, teat and glass in the hypochlorite solution (Milton), trapping the teat inside the glass.
Ensure that there are no bubbles of air inside the bottle.
Leave until the next feed (minimum time, two hours).
Drain, but do not rinse.

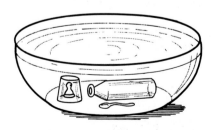

Sterilization of feeding utensils

Hypochlorite solution

This sterilizing solution should be renewed every twenty-four hours, and at a strength of one part solution in eighty of cold water. That is 15 ml ($\frac{1}{2}$ oz) to 1200 ml (2 pints) cold water.

The Milton container holds this amount.

As this solution corrodes metal all containers and spoons must be plastic, china or glass.

If boiling is carried out, the utensils are immersed in a large pan of warm water (again making sure that no bubbles of air remain).

Boil for three minutes.

Leave in the water until required.

It is important to thoroughly clean the utensils before sterilizing by either method; otherwise a film forms on the surface of the liquid and adequate sterilization cannot take place.

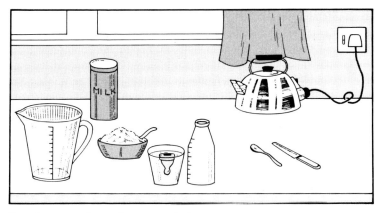

Requirements for making up a baby's feed

To prepare a feed

(1) *Requirements*

Milk
Sugar
Kettle of water (boiled)
Sterile jug and fork for mixing

Sterile bottle and spoon
Sterile teat and glass
Knife or tin opener as necessary

(2) *Method*

Clean the working surface
Spread a towel over the working surface
Collect utensils
Wash hands
Remove bottle from liquid and drain
Remove teat and place in the glass

(a) *If using cows' milk:*

Pour required volume of milk into the measuring jug.
Add equal quantity of water.
Add sugar and stir.
Pour into milk saucepan and bring to the boil.
Pour into the bottle.
Put on teat and cover with glass.
Allow to cool to correct temperature.

(b) *If using powdered milk:*

Put the required number of levelled scoops of powder into the measuring jug.
Add sugar, if required.
Pour on boiling water and mix with the spoon to a paste.
Make up to required amount with boiled water, whisking with a fork to prevent formation of lumps.
Pour into bottles and cover.

The teat

Care should be taken when putting the teat on the bottle to handle the rim only. Do not touch the part which will go into the baby's mouth. Cover the teat until the bottle is given to the baby.

Storage

Many mothers these days find it more convenient to make up a twenty-four hour supply of feeds. These should be

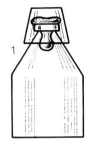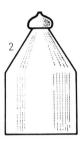

Storage of made-up feed   1 Inverted and covered teat   2 Valve

stored in a refrigerator with each individual bottle covered with a valve until required for use.

To give a feed

Place the bottle (with teat and cover in place) in a jug of hot water.
Change the baby's napkin.
Wash your hands.

Feeding a baby   1 Testing the temperature of a feed   2 Position for giving a feed

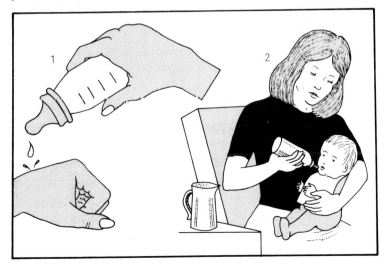

Sit on the most comfortable chair and support the baby as for breast feeding.

Shake a little milk on to the back of your hand to test that the mixture is warm – not hot.

Give the feed, making it as like breast feeding as possible.

Sleeping

The baby's cot is an important item. A carry cot is convenient as it can be carried everywhere and used day and night.

After a few weeks a larger cot will be necessary and a 4-foot drop-sided wooden cot is convenient.

The side-lowering mechanism should move easily but be sturdy. Cot bars should not be more than 7–8 cm apart otherwise the baby may put his head between them.

The mattress should be firm and protected by waterproof sheeting. Sheets should be either flannelette or cotton, not nylon. The cellular type of blankets are good. A pillow is unnecessary and dangerous.

Bathing a baby

Babies are so small and vulnerable that new mothers sometimes approach them with a little apprehension. Mothers should not be worried if they feel they have no natural maternal instinct; they need to get to know their baby, learn how to handle him, and develop assurance through practice. Help is needed in the early days, and this is the reason your health visitor will visit you after the midwife has safely helped you over the initial phase after the birth of the baby.

Requirements

A warm room, free of draughts (improvise a screen, if necessary, from a clothes horse and sheet)
Baby bath
Low chair
Trolley or table on which you place:
  baby cream
  baby powder

baby soap
Glass or plastic jar with cotton-wool swabs
Clean clothes (including nappy)
Safety pin
Large towel
Apron
Bucket for the soiled clothes
Paper bag for soiled swabs
Two face flannels (for the older baby)

Method

Prepare the room and collect everything you require.

Begin to fill the bath with cold water, adding hot until there is sufficient water at the right temperature. To make sure the temperature is right, put your elbow in the water. If it feels comfortable, it is correct (38°C or 100° F, just above blood heat).

Remove tops from jars and wash your own hands.

Undress the baby except for his napkin. Wrap him in the towel and wash his face very gently with a swab or soft flannel. Dry carefully.

Wash his head by laying him on your lap with his head towards the bath. Support his neck with your left hand, soap your right hand, wash and rinse his hair. Do not use soap every day but gently rinse with water on alternate days. Dry with the towel, using the flat of your hand so as not to damage the baby's fontanelle (a soft diamond shaped

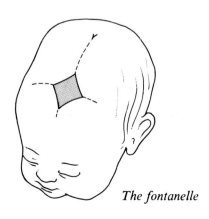

The fontanelle

area at the top of the head. There is also a smaller triangular area at the back of the head).

Remove the napkin, cleaning the buttocks with swabs if the baby has passed a stool. (By not removing the nappy until this stage you safeguard the face and eyes from infection). Lather your hands and soap the baby all over. Roll him on his side to soap his back. Immerse the baby in the bath. If you find him slippery when you lift, put him back on the towel and rinse and dry your own hands before lifting him into the bath.

To lift a baby into the bath, support his head and shoulders on your left hand and arm and lift his buttocks with your right hand.

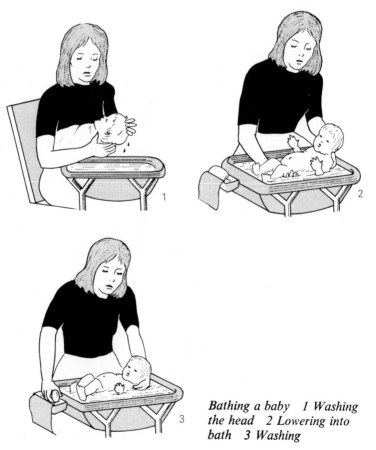

Bathing a baby   1 Washing the head   2 Lowering into bath   3 Washing

Still supporting the baby with your left hand and forearm, rinse off the soap with your right hand.

An older baby may sit up and play at this stage of his bath.

Lift the baby out of the bath and lay him face downwards on the towel. Dry his back.

Place the vest and prepared folded napkin in position. Turn the baby over on your lap, removing the towel as you do so. Dry the baby's front, sprinkle him with powder (if desired) and complete putting on his vest.

Cream his buttocks and fasten the napkin.

Put on the dress (making sure you don't touch his eyes as you put it over his head).

Place him in the cot, and clear away.

Sleep

A baby cannot distinguish night from day and will sleep twenty out of the twenty-four hours. He will awaken when he is uncomfortable or hungry. During the day, let him sleep in a cot or pram in the fresh air, if possible. Protect him by a cat net over the pram. Do not let the sun shine directly on to the baby. Make certain the brake is on the pram. Cold and wet weather do not matter so long as he is warm and protected from the elements. Do not put him out in fog. If there is no garden, keep the windows of his room wide open.

As the baby grows older, he requires less sleep. At six months he needs approximately eighteen hours, at twelve months about fifteen hours, and at two years, twelve to fourteen hours.

Sore buttocks

Redness and soreness of the buttocks can occur when nappies are not changed frequently enough, if the buttocks are not washed and dried carefully, or if the nappies have not been properly rinsed after washing.

Diarrhoea can also cause soreness. Whilst the baby is in his mother's uterus, his gut is full of a green sticky material called meconium. This is passed within a few hours of birth and continues for about three days when it becomes light brown in colour. This indicates that the milk he is taking is being digested and becoming mixed with the meconium. About the fourth or fifth day the stool becomes bright yellow and curd-like. Usually babies pass four to five stools in twenty-four hours, but breast-fed babies may pass fewer. Once weaning commences the stools become darker and firmer. If there is anything unusual about baby's stools, consult your doctor or health visitor.

Zinc and castor oil cream helps to protect the skin by providing a waterproof layer as well as soothing the soreness.

Laundering nappies

Wet nappies should be immersed in a pail of cold water as soon as they are removed.

Soiled nappies should be shaken over the lavatory, scrubbed under a running tap and soaked in cold water.

All nappies should be washed in hot water in a soap-flake solution. Soda should never be used. Thorough rinsing is essential.

If a washing machine with very hot water is used, no boiling is necessary.

Napisan is a chemical solution which cleanses and deodorizes nappies. They must be soaked for at least two hours, preferably overnight. Again, it is important to rinse thoroughly several times.

This method is quick, easy and economical.

Plastic and rubber pants should be used only on special occasions. They tend to make the baby hot and to encourage nappie-rash.

8. Nursing a sick child

Play and home

Play is an essential part of the life of a child. Through it he learns, develops and grows.

A baby plays with his fingers and toes; as he develops he explores his body: everything he handles becomes a plaything. This can be used to good advantage when he is ill. All activities – washing, eating, taking medicines – can be turned to play. This may mean giving up more of your time, but it makes an important contribution to a child's psychological development.

A child expects to be accepted, loved and liked – even more so when he is ill – and physical contact is most important.

The young patient should never be deceived. Questions should be answered honestly. When a child is given medicine he should be told it is medicine. If a pill or powder is offered in a spoonful of jam, he should be told why it is better for him to take it in this way. A child needs to feel secure, and must be able to trust the people around him at all times.

'Little pitchers have big ears' is an old, but not outdated, adage. Children are aware of everything that is going on around them and careless talk should be avoided: even if what you say is not particularly important, it may worry a child who will interpret it in his own way. 'Careless talk' can not only cause worry, but also sleeplessness, and fear.

Children are, by nature, truthful. Many live in a world of fantasy from time to time, but there is nothing unusual about that. In the course of normal mental development the world of fantasy will disappear.

It is as well to remember that sudden and dramatic changes can take place in the condition of a sick child. One minute he may be prostrate, listless, with a high fever: an hour or two later he may be sitting up and playing. Every change, and the time at which it occurs, should be noted, and reported to the family doctor on his next visit.

The nursing of a sick child calls for constant and intelligent observation and reporting. The correct treatment can very quickly produce the amazing recuperative power young people possess. Remember – they are very resilient.

General care of the sick child

It is important that the doctor's/nurse's instructions should be followed carefully. If there is anything you don't understand, ask. Make a note of what you want to ask, or report. If you wish to show a specimen to the doctor or nurse (e.g. a soiled nappy or vomit) it should be kept in the bathroom or lavatory and produced during their visit. Make sure there is a clean hand towel ready for the nurse's personal use.

If the ill child is taking medicines, keep them well out of his reach, and keep them cool (but not in a refrigerator unless instructed so to do). When pouring out medicines hold the bottle label side uppermost. This will keep the label clean – and the dosage instructions will remain legible. Throw all bottles away at the end of an illness.

Atmosphere

Whilst it is important to keep a firm, disciplined hold on the management of any illness, it is equally important that the child's routine is maintained in a homely atmosphere as much as possible, and that he is encouraged to keep up his spirits by substituting play for the activities he is missing.

Unless the doctor has specifically ordered that he should be kept in bed it is quite usual for a moderately sick child to be with the family – lying on a couch or on his mother's lap if he wishes. Follow his desires: he will tell you if he wants to go to bed: he will cease seeking your lap when he returns to normal health.

Put housework low on your list of priorities, but keep the child's room well aired, dusted and bright.

Sleeping

The child will know when he wants to go to sleep but, as far as possible, normal bedtimes should be kept. During an illness it is usually better (and more restful for everyone else) if the mother sleeps near her sick child so that she can more easily hear and deal with any calls during the night. A child with a very troublesome cough may find it more comfortable to sleep sitting up supported by pillows. A child under the age of two who has a severe cough may find it comforting to be held propped up in his parent's arms whilst trying to get to sleep.

Washing and going to the lavatory

Often it is far easier for the child to use a pot instead of going to the lavatory. He can then stay in an even temperature, and it also enables specimens of his motion or water to be kept. It is important that handwashing is carried out before eating and after 'potting' (this, of course, applies not only in the case of illness, but also when good health is enjoyed). Do not give aperients (medicines to induce opening of the bowels) unless ordered to do so.

A sick child's bed should be made at least once a day and a change of bedclothes and night clothes helps a feverish, sick child feel fresher and more comfortable.

Tidy and smooth the bed for comfort but do not be too fussy about its appearance.

Washing and hair brushing should be carried out at least twice a day (in the morning and before settling down for the night). If the child has a fever, sponging with warm water will bring some relief.

Teeth should be brushed regularly, as usual, with extra brushing or mouthwashings after being sick. If the child is likely to vomit, keep a clean, covered bowl within his reach. When he is being sick, stay with him.

If a child over the age of three has an irritating rash, allow him to dab calamine lotion on to his skin: it will help prevent scratching.

The common cold

This may be caused by one of many viruses. The symptoms are known to us all – redness and soreness of the throat, sneezing, and an outpouring of nasal discharge. At first this discharge is clear and watery but, when invaded by bacteria, it becomes thick and turns yellow or yellowish green.

Sometimes this catarrh trickles down the back of the throat, irritates the back of the mouth and causes the child to cough. Because this 'drip' is encouraged by the horizontal position, the cough becomes worse when the child is lying down, i.e. at night. If it settles in the lungs, it can set off bronchitis (inflammation of the tubes of the lung) or pneumonia. It is therefore advisable to nurse the young patient in a sitting-up position.

Because the Eustachian tube (the tube which runs from the back of the mouth to the ear) in small babies is short and straight, they often develop a 'pink ear' as a complication of a cold. This is inflammation of the middle ear (otitis media) of which there are many forms and degrees of severity (see p. 103).

Nursing care

Most children prefer to be up and about unless very feverish. It is wise, however, to keep a child indoors if he is running a temperature. If he runs around the house, he may sweat. This is not harmful, but if fluid is lost it must be replaced, so make sure that he drinks a lot: hot sweet drinks can be soothing.

A simple linctus may be given to ease a troublesome cough at night but, as yet, there is no cure for the common cold. Even the giving of aspirin has its opponents. Although aspirin brings down the temperature temporarily, by decreasing natural resistance to the disease, it increases the risk of secondary infection.

If this occurs, the physician may prescribe antibiotics.

Allergic rhinitis

This is inflammation of the nose caused by an allergy to a substance. Children who appear always to 'have a cold' may be suffering from allergic rhinitis.

When exposed to certain irritants, such as pollen or cats' hairs, some people – adults as well as children – react by developing a non-infectious inflammation.

When an allergic reaction occurs in the lining of the nose, it is called allergic rhinitis; when the skin reacts, an urticaria results; the eyes develop an allergic conjunctivitis (inflammation of the lining of the eyes) and so on. There is usually no fever associated with allergic rhinitis. The nasal discharge may be thin and watery, or thick and mucoid (like mucus). The eyes often water.

Treatment

Some drugs given for the treatment of allergies are called antihistamines. Antihistamines should not be given without medical advice. In fact, given as nose drops or ointments, they themselves can cause allergy. A doctor's prescription should always be procured, even though many such medicines can be obtained without one.

Otitis media

The ear is divided – structurally and functionally – into three parts: external, middle and inner. Inflammation of the ear is known as otitis, inflammation of the middle ear as otitis media.

The external ear includes the ear lobe and the canal leading to the eardrum. Behind the drum is a small cavity.

The middle ear contains three small bones called malleus, incus and stapes. These transmit vibrations to the fluid canals which lie in the *inner ear*. Nerves carrying the sensations of hearing and balance travel from the inner ear to the brain.

Boils sometimes occur in the outer ear (otitis externa). These can be very painful but need not give cause for anxiety.

Because the inner ear is virtually sealed off from outside sources of infection, otitis interna is rare.

Infection can spread rapidly to the middle ear which is connected by the Eustachian tube to the mouth and the nasal cavity.

Inflammation of the middle ear produces catarrh-like fluid which may be sterile or infected. Pressure of this fluid on the eardrum can cause it to perforate. Also, the three

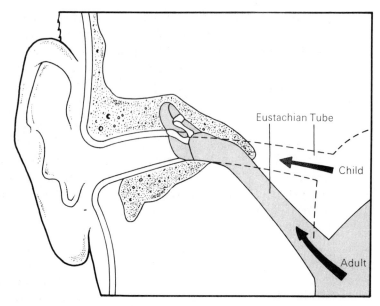

How infection reaches the middle ear

small bones then cannot function normally and hearing may be affected.

Acute otitis media is very common in children under the age of five. The commonest symptom is earache. If it is not treated, the drum may perforate and, if damaged by frequent past attacks, the first sign of this may be a fluid discharge.

Infection of the mastoid bone (just beyond the middle ear) can be serious because it leads directly to the brain. Before the advent of antibiotics many children with mastoiditis had to undergo surgery to prevent the development of a brain abscess. Unfortunately, this often damaged hearing.

Whilst modern treatment has lowered the hazard of mastoiditis and the formation of brain abscesses, the problem of persistent middle ear catarrh remains. It is usually painless, but hearing is impaired. It is for this reason that medical advice should be sought at once if a child's hearing is thought to be affected after an attack of otitis media.

To test the hearing of a child, stand behind him, gently close each ear in turn with your finger and ask the child to repeat the words you whisper to him. Words of a similar sound used as consonants are the hardest to hear, e.g. dish, fish, wish: cat, rat, mat: horse, course, force.

Nursing care

Treatment will be ordered by the family doctor. Sometimes antibiotics may be prescribed. Ear drops to relieve pain must be used judiciously as they can damage the ear drum. (See Chapter 6 for the instillation of ear drops). Small doses of a pain-killing drug may be given if the child is kept awake by pain. Paracetamol is often prescribed for this purpose.

Conjunctivitis

This is inflammation of the eyelid and the mucous membrane covering the white of eye, and is one of the commonest infections of babies and young children. It can be caused by several different bacteria. The eye becomes red, and often there is pus inside the sac of the eye. Conjunctivitis is highly contagious. The infected child should have his own face flannel and towel.

Medical advice should always be sought but, pending a visit to the family doctor, the eye may be bathed and the pus gently swabbed using warm water which has been boiled and allowed to cool. Swab from the nose outwards, using each swab once only. Inflammation of the eye from any cause whatsoever should be treated by a doctor.

Influenza

Influenza is an acute infection caused by a virus and accompanied by a fever. There are three main types of virus – A, B and C. Each has sub-types – Ab, Az, etc. and each has its own immunity response, so that an attack from one virus does not give immunity to another.

The extent of an epidemic varies according to the number of people immune to the particular virus rampant. Because epidemics 'travel in waves around the world' their path can usually be pre-plotted, and preventive measures taken by the government of each country.

The onset of influenza is very rapid. Fever and general malaise are the first symptoms. The throat and eyelids often become red and sore, whilst the whole chest feels 'raw' inside. The wind pipe is most severely affected and pneumonia can be an added complication.

Without complications, the fever lasts for four to eight days; the temperature often falling to normal after the first two or three days, and then rising again.

Nursing care

The greatest problem when nursing a child who has flu is in keeping him amused. He will probably feel more comfortable in bed. His fluid intake should be kept up: glucosed fruit juices and squashes are particularly soothing to a sore throat.

Pain killing and temperature-lowering medicines such as aspirin or paracetamol should only be given if prescribed by the family physician. Some doctors believe it best not to interfere with the body's own natural defence against infection, that is, they believe the fever should not be attacked, but left to burn itself out.

If the temperature rises above 40°C (104°F) and remains at that point for twelve hours or longer, the doctor should be asked to call.

A close watch should be kept on the child's breathing and, if there is any difficulty, or any sign of blueness of the skin, the doctor should be informed at once.

If there are complications of influenza they are usually treated with prescribed antibiotics.

Influenza vaccine

The vaccine which has been produced over recent years contains a mixture of antigens (immunity producing substances) from various strains of virus.

The most serious influenza epidemics are usually those caused by a new strain, and the World Influenza Centre collects viruses from all new outbreaks in an attempt to prepare modified vaccines against new strains. A vaccine which can be taken by mouth is also being tested.

Tonsilitis

Throat infections are often localized, affecting only the tonsils which may be inflamed, and swollen, or covered with patches of exudate.

If the infection spreads outside the tonsil a peritonsillar abscess will develop (quinsy).

There is fever, difficulty and pain in swallowing, and enlargement and tenderness of glands of the neck at the angles of the jaw. In quinsy there is also difficulty in opening the mouth.

Most attacks of tonsilitis usually respond well to penicillin and it is no longer a serious illness. However, if frequent attacks occur some surgeons advocate removal of the tonsils. In children the operation is usually combined with removal of the adenoids and attention to any middle ear discharge.

Infectious hepatitis

Infectious hepatitis and serum hepatitis are both caused by a virus.

Infectious hepatitis is carried in the faeces: it may spread by direct contact where there is poor hygiene or it may be water- or food-borne. Serum hepatitis is conveyed by blood. The virus enters the bloodstream either during blood transfusion or any injection where a trace of the infected blood remains in the needle of the syringe. For example, drug addicts who share syringes are vulnerable.

Disposable syringes should be used whenever possible.

Incubation periods

The incubation period of infectious hepatitis is about one month; of serum hepatitis, about three months.

The onset is gradual with abdominal discomfort and 'tummy upset'. The urine becomes dark (with bile) and the conjunctivae (whites of the eyes) yellow. The jaundice spreads all over the body. General malaise lasts for a week or so but the yellowness may persist for several weeks.

Hepatitis must never be regarded as a minor illness. It is one of the most severe infections and causes much debility. If it is not cured, it can result in coma and death.

Treatment

The main treatment is rest, not necessarily confinement to bed, but the patient should be encouraged to 'take things easy'. Long convalescence is essential.

Diet restriction is not necessary. The main aim is to keep the patient well-nourished. During the first week he will probably have little appetite. He may dislike fatty food for a few weeks. Judicial use of drugs is important because some drugs – hypnotics for example – are toxic to the liver.

Gastro-enteritis

Like the acute form occurring in babies, this condition causes frequent sickness and loose motions. Acute diarrhoea, with or without vomiting, is common. Most travellers suffer 'a tummy upset' – whether journeying from or to the UK. Sometimes the cause is identifiable as a particular type of bacteria carried by dirty hands, flies or water. More often than not, no cause can be found, and the infection is blamed on a 'virus going around' or, if abroad, 'the local water'.

To determine whether a virus is responsible, special tests are necessary as simple bacteriological examination of stools does not identify the type of organism.

Nursing care

Stop all food and encourage the drinking of clear fluids. If the diarrhoea is only mild, the child's normal activity need be only slightly curtailed.

If it is severe, there is a grave danger of dehydration, and the small patient must be encouraged to drink plenty of watery fluids. Severe dehydration can be recognized by loss of elasticity of the skin. Gentle pinching together of the skin of the abdomen will demonstrate this. All soiled garments –

bedding, napkins, etc. – must be thoroughly washed and sterilized (by boiling when possible).

When nursing a child suffering from sickness and diarrhoea hands must be carefully washed and dried after each service given. Disposable towels have an obvious advantage.

No food (not even milk) should be given for twenty-four hours. To keep up the essential supply of salt, add a pinch to each glass of water, disguising the taste by adding fruit juice or sugar.

If there is severe loss of other minerals, the family doctor may prescribe special tablets containing these.

When there has been no diarrhoea or vomiting for twenty-four hours, half strength milk may be given, gradually increasing the fluid diet to a light diet and finally to normal meals.

Anti-diarrhoea mixtures are available and may relieve the symptoms, especially colic. Plain kaolin is available without a doctor's prescription but if symptoms continue, a doctor's advice should be obtained. He will decide whether or not antibiotics are necessary.

Remember that most cases of infectious diarrhoea clear up by withholding food and encouraging the drinking of fluids.

Coeliac disease

This disease becomes apparent soon after weaning a child on to foods with flour which contains gluten. The child's gut reacts to wheat protein in such a way that damages the mucose and thus reduces its ability to absorb necessary foodstuffs. There is offensive diarrhoea, and fatigue due to anaemia (iron and folic acid are not absorbed). Other symptoms are mouth ulcers, loss of appetite, loss of weight, distension and wind.

Treatment is a strict gluten-free diet for life.

The Coeliac Society, run by patients for patients, provides very useful information – and some valuable hints on how to make the necessary strict diet interesting.

All forms of flour must be omitted; wheat and rye should be excluded from the diet. Some patients also have to avoid oats and barley.

Meat, fish, eggs, cheese, milk, fruit and vegetables may be eaten but not with gravy (if thickened with flour) or sauce. Food must not be coated with butter or breadcrumbs. Fats, sugar, jams and boiled sweets may be eaten.

It should be remembered that bread substitutes such as Ryvita, Energen rolls, cakes and biscuits all contain flour. Special bread and rusks are available but many people prefer to do their own gluten-free baking.

9. Some disorders and problems of childhood and adolescence

Some problems and disorders of childhood
Bedwetting

There is wide variation in the development of children. Usually a baby under the age of fourteen-fifteen months has no control of his bladder. He will train himself to become dry somewhere between eighteen months and two and a half years.

Boys are sometimes slower than girls to gain bladder control because they have a smaller capacity (their bladders are smaller). Encourage, but do not force, 'clean habits'. Your attitude is all important if phobias are to be avoided. Be matter-of-fact, and never bribe. Sometimes a 'bad habit' is re-introduced by an older child when a new baby arrives in the family as, in this way, the older child finds it receives more attention. A little reassurance and extra affection will often cure the trouble quickly.

Most children are dry at night by the age of three, allowing for the occasional accident, of course. After the age of five, bedwetting at night is regarded as a problem and is called nocturnal enuresis. This may run in families and may right itself by the age of ten without any treatment being given.

Occasionally it persists into adult life.

Children do not wet their beds on purpose: they dislike it as much as their parents. Although you may find it troublesome, involving extra washing, ruined mattresses and unpleasant smells, never scold or punish.

Some children who have unusually small and sensitive bladders find it difficult to gain control, and some training may be helpful. Give the child plenty of fluids during the day and encourage him to wait five–ten minutes beyond the time he first feels the need to empty his bladder.

There can be a medical reason for enuresis, such as a mild infection or a slight structural deformity and, therefore, if bedwetting persists it is wise to consult the family doctor.

Only if such medical reasons are ruled out, is home management the most important way of helping. A sense of security is essential, because emotions such as jealousy, excitement, insecurity (brought about by admission to hospital or visits away from home) may produce enuresis.

The child's bedroom should be warm and well ventilated. Make sure he has a night-light or torch so that he is able to find his way to the lavatory quickly and easily. Keep the mattress protected – a fitted waterproof cover is best for older children and rubber sheeting for younger. See that sheets and pyjamas are made of drip-dry material.

The parents' attitude is vital. Parents must convince the child that they understand the problem and are there to help him. They must make it perfectly clear that they, do not love him less because he wets the bed. A sensitive child can very easily feel rejected and become anxious and unhappy. Encourage him, build up his confidence, but do not overdo the 'rewards'. Often they increase the anxiety.

A special electric alarm device for nocturnal enuresis may be bought or loaned from school clinics. It consists of a buzzer which is placed under the bottom sheet and which rings as soon as it becomes the slightest bit damp. The child soon becomes trained to wake before the bell rings. And this is certainly worth a few nights' broken sleep on the part of the rest of the family, because it usually does work after a week or so.

But, whatever help is given, or taken, with sensible and sympathetic management, and eradication of the root cause, nocturnal enuresis can almost always be cured.

Undescended testes

The testes develop from primitive cells in the abdomen and descend during development through the inguinal canal to lie in the scrotum. In some infants the testes may not be down in the right place, due to a defect of the testes or the mechanical interruption of its descent. The testes will develop normal spermatozoa (the seeds of the male necessary to fertilize the egg of the female) if they lie in the scrotum. If retained in the abdomen, sterility will result.

A boy with undescended testes may be treated before puberty with the injection of a substance called chorionic gonadotrophin to try to stimulate descent. If this fails, surgery will be needed.

Habits

Babies and young children sometimes develop habits which, although unimportant, worry their parents. Most will disappear in time.

Thumbsucking

The greatest danger with thumbsucking, if it persists for too long, is that it may alter the shape of the mouth and teeth. Otherwise it does little harm.

A breast-fed baby is less likely to become a thumbsucker than a bottle-fed baby because the former often goes on sucking after the milk supply is exhausted. With a bottle-fed baby the bottle is taken away as soon as the milk is finished. Quite rightly so, as if the baby sucks in air it will only give him colic. But it does mean he goes short of the action of sucking which gives him not only food but also pleasure and comfort. So he resorts to his thumb.

There are two schools of thought about allowing babies to have a dummy or a piece of clean muslin to suck. If you decide to allow your baby to have a dummy, do make sure it is the right shape and *never* dip it in sugar or milk or, indeed, into anything at all. A pleasant taste will protract the desire to suck, as well as having a disastrous effect on teeth!

Head banging

This habit usually develops about the age of eighteen months. The baby bangs his head against the wall before going to sleep. This usually happens when he is *over*-tired. Again, it is a method of obtaining some kind of comfort and getting relief from tension.

Other children roll their heads from side to side or beat their heads with their fists. Even more common is cot-

shifting. The child will kneel on all fours and by bouncing – in rhythm, from which he derives comfort – will move his cot across the room.

Sometimes there is a physical reason – such as earache or teething – for these habits, but often the cause is psychological. You may be trying to make him grow up too quickly, or arranging too strict a routine. This is particularly so with first babies whose parents are over-anxious. Remember that worry is 'catching' and that a harassed parent can often affect her baby in this way.

Never scold a child for producing one of these 'nervous habits'. It will make matters worse. Don't tie him down in his cot or frustrate him in any way. If he is in danger of hurting himself, pad the cot sides with a blanket. But the best treatment is to create a happy, relaxed atmosphere – especially at bedtime.

If any of these habits persist, consult your health visitor or family doctor.

Handling the genitals

It is not dirty or wrong for a young child to handle his genitals and he should not be scolded or spanked for doing so. Punishment may do untold harm and affect his sexual life later on.

Young children explore their genitals as they examine their fingers and toes – it is natural curiosity.

Many older children masturbate – without realizing what they are doing – merely because it gives them pleasure. This is a passing phase (unless it is prolonged by a shocked attitude on the part of the parents), and the child should not be punished.

Usually children masturbate when frightened by secret or imagined fears. They derive comfort from this 'sensation'.

It is certainly wrong to tell children they will die, go mad, or become ill if they handle their genitals. It is, however, necessary to find out why a child does so. Has he plenty of playmates? Is he jealous of a new brother or sister? Are you pushing him at school? Do you talk 'O' levels at him? Is he competing with older, brighter, children? Are you making too much of his school successes (or failures)? Have you for some reason (e.g. because you now go out to work) cut down on the time you give him?

Children need to be wanted and loved. Tell them they are, and show them, too. But don't let them know you are worried about this 'habit'. It will only increase tension and prolong the phase.

Provided you have checked with your doctor that there is no physical cause, give your child emotional security and love – and ignore the habit. It will disappear in time.

Infections

Worms
Threadworm

In this country the most common type of worm is threadworm. This is particularly so in young children, although whole families may be affected.

The chief symptom is anal pruritis (irritation around and inside the anus). This is because the female is laying her eggs in this area.

Diagnosis is made by detecting ova (eggs) on a piece of sellotape applied to the skin around the anus first thing in the morning.

Effective treatment is carried out with piperazine. Reinfection should be prevented by careful handwashing, especially after bowel action, and before meals. Nails should be cut short.

Tapeworm

Segments of the worms are passed in the stools. It is a fairly common condition in this country.

Treatment is the administration of niclosamide.

Fasting must take place before two tablets of 500 mg are chewed with a little water. Another two tablets are given a little later.

This treatment is very effective and there are no side effects.

Head lice and nits

Most mothers believe their children will never have lice and nits, but it is true that the number of reported cases in the UK in recent years has been increasing.

Lice can be picked up in schools, colleges, cinemas, buses and trains: indeed, in any public place. If a child becomes infected, it does not mean that his parents and home are dirty! It is a condition which can very easily be picked up, and passed on, and because of this an infection can run through an entire school very quickly.

The louse is the insect; the nit, the egg it lays. The eggs, which are about ·32 cm long, are more easily seen than the lice. When lice lay their eggs they secrete a very sticky substance and this fixes the nits very firmly to strands of hair. When the baby louse is hatched it leaves behind its grey 'shell', which can easily be mistaken for dandruff. Unlike dandruff, however, it cannot be 'shed' as it is stuck firmly to the hair.

Lice cause irritation and if the child scratches he can cause an infection of the scalp resulting in patches of sore skin and swollen neck glands. Nits can be treated successfully by various insecticides such as Derbac or Lorexene lotions, and Derbac shampoo or soap will help to prevent a recurrence.

These lotions must be applied correctly if they are to be successful, so follow the maker's instructions carefully. After treatment, inspect the hair daily using a fine toothcomb. Part the hair in a number of small partings and comb the hair from the scalp to the tip.

As infection is very easily spread, brushes and combs, hats, caps and scarves should be treated – i.e. washed, cleaned, disinfected, and kept separate from those belonging to other members of the family.

Acne vulgaris

Acne is a disorder of the sweat glands and hair roots.

This condition, which can take the form of blackheads, red papules, pustules, nodules and scarring, begins soon after puberty has been reached.

The tendency to acne disappears after a variable number of years but during those years it can cause much mental distress. This, and the resulting scars, justify treatment.

Excessive greasiness of the skin can be dealt with by washing the affected area with an antiseptic soap such as Cidal, or an antiseptic lotion such as Phisolox. Sulphur paste BPC induces peeling of the skin, and ultra-violet light is helpful for some young people. Your family doctor should be consulted.

If there is associated dandruff, a medicated shampoo should be used regularly and brushes and combs kept scrupulously clean.

Hay fever

This is one of our most common diseases. It is an allergy affecting about 10 per cent of the population of the UK and its symptoms range in severity from trivial attacks of sneezing to life-threatening attacks of asthma. Grass pollen is by far the most common cause of hay fever in the UK.

Severe hay fever and asthma can occur directly during or after exposure to grass pollen. Patients can do themselves harm by repeatedly exposing themselves to conditions to which they are allergic. Whilst pollen cannot be avoided altogether, the following precautions should be taken by any member of the family who suffers from hay fever.

1. Never walk through long grass.
2. Sleep with bedroom windows closed during May, June and July.
3. Do not go for holidays or outings in the country, or camp during these months.
4. Travel by train or car should be undertaken with the windows closed during May–July.
5. If injection treatment is given, observe the above for the three years of its duration.

Antihistamine drugs may control mild hay fever.

Corticosteroid drugs must be prescribed by a doctor and used only as a last resort, because of side effects.

Desensitization is probably the best approach where adequate symptomatic relief is difficult to obtain. Great care must always be taken because over-dosage with pollen antigen is extremely dangerous. The treatment must be begun in January or February and finished before the pollen is in the air i.e. April (or early May at the latest).

The young adolescent

Painful periods

Victorian mothers gave much advice to their daughters concerning their periods. During these days they were not allowed to bath, wash their hair, get their feet wet, drink cold fluids, or eat cold food. Times have changed!

Menstruation is not an illness, and a welcome result of the change in attitude is that discomfort has become less because we do not expect it to be so great. Certainly, periods are often inconvenient, but if they are also painful something should be done about it.

The medical name for painful periods is dysmenorrhoea: even that is not a complaint – it is a symptom, and the cause of the symptom should be sought.

Let us consider the process of menstruation briefly. Each girl baby is born with thousands of egg cells in the ovaries. These lie dormant until puberty when hormones are secreted and the eggs 'ripen'. Once a month – mid-cycle – one egg is expelled, and passes down the fallopian tube to the womb (uterus). During this time the lining of the womb becomes thicker and blood containing oxygen and food for a fertilized egg cell is stored. If fertilization occurs, the egg imbeds itself in the lining of the womb and a baby develops. If fertilization does not occur, the lining breaks down and the extra blood, plus the unfertilized egg cell, are expelled – as menstrual flow, or the 'period'. This action continues monthly, except during pregnancy, until the 'change of life' (menopause). All this should happen easily, regularly, and without pain.

Pain can be caused by congestion of the organs, holding up the flow. Constipation and lack of exercise are two important and common causes. Sometimes too much starchy food and too little fruit and vegetables cause constipation: a balanced diet and plenty of fluids is essential to health.

When a slight obstruction holds up the flow, a minor operation (dilatation and curettage) will widen the cervical canal (the passage from uterus to vagina). However, this usually rights itself after sexual intercourse and child-bearing.

Very sensitive nerve endings in the uterus can be treated surgically or by drugs. Sometimes the administration of hormones will increase a scanty flow – but this should never be attempted without a doctor's prescription.

Anaemia may also be the cause of a scanty flow but, again, the advice of your family doctor must be sought, for there are many forms of anaemia which can only be diagnosed by blood tests.

Adequate sleep, fresh air and mental and physical activity are very important. And for those who are unable to take exercise in the form of walking, tennis, swimming, etc. early morning exercises can be a reasonable substitute.

Vaginal discharges

Vaginal discharges are very common and have many causes. They do not necessarily signify cancer or venereal disease.

In a healthy female there is always a vaginal secretion. At certain times there is more secretion than at others: just before a period and half-way through the period cycle when an egg cell is released from the ovary. Also during pregnancy. This secretion should be clear and inoffensive. It keeps the membrane moist and, because of its slight antiseptic effect, free of many germs.

A white discharge, in excess of normal, is known as 'the whites' (leucorrhoea) and looks like milk. This often occurs when a woman is run down, suffering from physical or mental stress, debilitated, or recovering from illness. It can also be caused by a faulty diet, and very often a well-balanced diet, fresh air, exercise and adequate sleep puts things right very quickly. Because the glands which produce hormones have not settled into a proper rhythm 'the whites' is common during adolescence. Again, with attention to diet, rest and exercise, this will quickly right itself.

119

If the vaginal discharge is profuse, thick, frothy, offensive or coloured, the family doctor's advice should be sought. There are many common infections which may be the cause. One is monilia (it also causes thrush in babies' mouths); another, trichomonas. These cause irritation but, with medical treatment, can be completely cured.

Sometimes a polypus, a small wart-like growth (which, by the way, has nothing to do with cancer) in the cervix (the neck of the womb), may bleed or become infected. This is easily removed, so the doctor's advice should be sought.

Inflammation of this channel between the vagina and uterus is called cervicitis and produces an offensive discharge which is a mixture of mucus and pus (mucopurulent). This is usually accompanied by other symptoms such as fatigue, headache and, sometimes, backache. The family doctor should be consulted.

Sexually transmitted diseases

Because sexual intercourse outside marriage is prevalent, this generation has produced many illegitimate babies, and the number of cases of venereal disease has increased.

Venereal diseases are infectious and are transmitted by sexual intercourse. There are two main varieties – gonorrhoea and syphilis. Because each can have very serious long-term effects, medical advice must be sought. Venereal disease cannot be cured without treatment, *even though the symptoms may disappear.* If the condition is neglected, irreparable damage can be done to health – and to the next generation. If treated in its early stages, venereal disease can be cured. If treatment is too long delayed sterility, paralysis, blindness and insanity can result.

Syphilis

The first sign of syphilis appears two – six weeks after infection, in the form of a small, painless sore on or around the sexual organs. This disappears and is replaced by a widespread rash, and sometimes additional sore areas. The disappearance of the original sore sometimes causes

120

the young man or woman to think the infection has cleared up and they are lulled into a false sense of security. Such a disappearance does not signify cure, but rather the end of the first stage of the infection.

Gonorrhoea

First symptoms of this disease occur within a few days of infection. There is inflammation, a discharge, and pain is experienced on passing water. Often these symptoms are only mild but, if neglected, the infection spreads internally.

Qualified medical advice should be sought immediately. Special clinics attached to hospitals where nurses and doctors can be consulted in privacy may be preferred to the family doctor. Information concerning the patient is not divulged to his family unless written consent is given.

It is impossible to diagnose venereal disease without a blood test. The result of this can be known in half an hour and treatment can begin with the minimum of delay.

Prevention of venereal diseases

It is the duty of every parent to tell his child about venereal disease: how it is caught; how to avoid getting it; what to do if one does get it. Early advice and treatment is essential. Staff of these special clinics of genito-urinary medicine do not moralize or preach. If you suspect a young adolescent in your care of having a venereal disease, seek medical advice immediately. At least one life is at stake, and, if treated in the early stages, the disease can be cured.

Drug addiction

Misuse of drugs

The misuse of drug substances is international. It may be the use of 'pep pills' (amphetamines), strong alcohol, marijuana and LSD or glue-sniffing.

It was not this generation, but the one before – certainly in the UK at any rate – who misused pep pills. Twenty years ago many general practitioners were prescribing them for their obese, depressed and unhappy patients. This practice was widespread. Certainly relief from stress is obtained from their use, and among a group of people 'reefers' provide a 'sharing' feeling which family life is unable to offer them. Divorced parents, wars, hi-jackings, strikes, fathers made redundant, and bombs (as well as college, sex and 'growing up') add up to a formidable list of turmoils which many young people have to face before reaching maturity. Is it any wonder that they seek 'props'?

The adolescent needs protection from the drug hazard prevalent in today's society. We know that long-term drug misuse brings personality deterioration, and that an already unstable personality can be precipitated into mental illness.

Unfortunately there are families where mutual trust and confidence between generations is missing. Open discussion can often reduce the stresses and strains on both sides. Parents must listen as well as talk! (See Chapter 16 for Addictions.)

10. Nursing a patient with an infectious illness

Illness has many different causes: it may be the result of an accident, malfunction of organs, or disease. In the UK, during the last century, the incidence of diseases due to infection has decreased because of improved living standards and the production of vaccines and sera to prevent them.

Serious infectious diseases are still common in primitive countries and in some developing countries, where standards of housing, nutrition and hygiene are not so high as in the UK.

Bacteria are present everywhere. When these minute living organisms enter the body they have one of three effects. They can be:

1. harmless – or even beneficial – to the body;
2. harmful – but the body defences overcome them;
3. harmful – and cause disease.

If these bacteria spread from one person to another, the disease so caused is termed 'infectious'.

Infectious diseases have certain characteristics in common:

(i) an incubation period (the time between the entrance of bacteria to the body and the appearance of signs and symptoms). This varies from a few days in the case of scarlet fever and diptheria, to two weeks or more in the case of German measles or mumps.

(ii) an early phase of illness, called the invasive prodromal stage (the same signs and symptoms appear in all patients but vary in severity).

Many infectious diseases produce a rash and may give rise to complications.

Any child with a fever persisting longer than twenty-four hours, or who comes out in a rash, should be seen by a doctor.

How an infectious disease is spread

Direct contact

Bacteria can travel from one person to another by direct contact. In this way, a family or an entire school or community can be infected. People who harbour and pass on bacteria without being ill themselves are called 'carriers'.

Droplet infection

Air leaving the nose and mouth contains water vapour and bacteria. If this air is breathed in by another person (in an ill-ventilated room, for instance) infection may follow.

Fomites

These are articles such as books, handkerchiefs, etc., which have been handled or used by the infected person. Other people handling or using them may, in turn, become infected.

Infected food

Bacteria can be present on food. If infected food is eaten it can cause intestinal infection. Milk and water can also act as carriers of infection.

Vectors

Insects carry bacteria and some infect by puncturing the skin and discharging parasites into the blood stream, i.e.,

How infection spreads   1 Droplet infection – coughing   2 Excreta as source – lavatory   3 Dust as source – sweeping

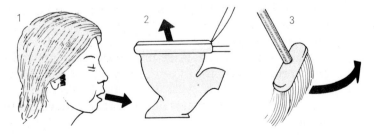

mosquitoes. Flies also carry bacteria from infected material to food and fluids.

Care of a patient suffering from an infectious disease

When nursing a patient with an infectious disease there are two main aspects of care to be borne in mind:

1. the care of the patient.
2. the prevention of the spread of the disease to others and to yourself.

The care of the patient varies according to the disease and its severity. A child with German measles may be only slightly 'off colour', whilst an adult with smallpox can be very seriously ill.

Various lines can be taken to prevent the spread of disease. In the case of infectious diseases of childhood few preventive measures are taken, sometimes none at all: but a patient with a serious infection which may prove fatal, or result in a complication such as partial paralysis, is nursed in isolation.

When barrier nursing is conducted the patient should be confined to one room. Personal contact is restricted, visitors wear gowns and masks for protection, and eating, drinking and personal toilet utensils are kept for the patient's sole use.

Barrier nursing

If the doctor asks you to 'barrier nurse' the patient, this is what you should do:

1. *Practise isolation*

If possible, the patient should be nursed in a room on his own.

Every visitor and attendant must don a gown or overall on entering the room and remove it on leaving. If the infection is droplet-carried masks must also be worn.

Attendants may wear rubber gloves. If not, hands must be washed very carefully immediately after tending or visiting the patient.

Disposable equipment and protective covering must be burnt.

125

2. *Prevent droplet infection*

Paper handkerchiefs should be used, collected in a paper bag after use and then burnt.

Coughs and sneezes should be controlled into a handkerchief.

Windows should be kept open. (If necessary, screens should be placed around the bed to prevent draughts.)

3. *Prevent the rest of the family becoming infected*

All books, magazines, toys, toilet requisites, etc., must be kept for the patient's exclusive use.

China, glass and cutlery should be put on one side and kept separate from the rest of the household supply. After use, it should be washed and boiled for five minutes (in a fish kettle or large saucepan.) This pan, a dishcloth and a tea-towel should be used exclusively for the patient's utensils.

All washing and toilet requisites should be kept in the patient's room.

Soiled bedlinen should be taken straight from the patient's room and laundered independently of the family wash. If it is not possible to do this at home the linen must be soaked in disinfectant before sending it to the laundrette or laundry. (Those disinfectants recommended for babies' nappies are eminently suitable for this job also.)

All magazines, books and newspapers must be burnt after being handled by an infected patient. Infected library books should be wrapped in plastic disinfecting, sealed and returned to the library with an explanation. This ensures that appropriate measures will be taken by the authorities.

If you are buying toys for infected children they should be cheap and 'burnable', or of a substance which can be boiled.

4. *Prevent infection by excreta*

Bedpans and urinals should be emptied immediately after use and the contents flushed away at once.

Disinfectants should be used liberally to cover the excreta and to disinfect the utensils. Seek guidance from the doctor or nurse.

5. *Prevent infection by food*

Small helpings of food should be served at frequent intervals and any uneaten portions burnt immediately. All food must be covered and never left exposed to flies. Fly repellants should be used in the sick room, but kept well away from food.

6. *When the patient has recovered*

When the period of infection is over the patient should bath and have his hair washed.

Sometimes pillows and mattress need to be fumigated and your doctor or nurse will tell you how to arrange this. If this is not necessary put them out into the air and sun for several hours.

Blankets and linen should be washed and dried out-of-doors.

The sick room should be washed and cleaned thoroughly and the windows left open for several hours.

Airing a room and bedding.

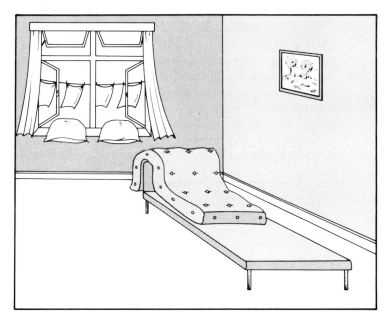

Immunity

Infectious diseases, then, are spread by individuals; by air and dust; by infected food, water and milk; by flies and rats; and by infected articles such as bedlinen, toys and books.

But just because a person is exposed to germs which cause a disease this does not mean that he will necessarily develop it. In fact, only a few people exposed to an infection may get the disease. Some people develop an immunity to it. Good food, drugs and immunization can help the body resist infection.

Immunity is the power of resistance of the body against disease and especially against germs or their poisonous products (toxins). The body has many ways of protecting itself, one being that when a patient recovers from an infectious disease he invariably becomes immune to it. This means that the body has formed certain substances (antibodies) which, in the future, will prevent the germ of that disease from having any further harmful effect. This is an 'acquired' or 'active' immunity. It may be temporary: it may last a lifetime. Few people contract whooping cough, chicken pox or mumps more than once, because the immunity usually lasts a lifetime.

Immunity may be obtained in various other ways. A new-born baby derives immunity to certain diseases such as measles or chicken pox from his mother, if she has had those diseases. This 'inherited immunity' explains why babies rarely develop measles or chicken pox during the first few months of life even when exposed to older brothers and sisters who are infected.

Sometimes people have a very slight attack of an infectious disease which may pass almost unnoticed. This will nevertheless produce antibodies which will protect them against further attacks of that particular disease.

Immunization may also be obtained by vaccination and inoculation.

Vaccination and Inoculation

Vaccination offers a protection against smallpox.

The vaccine is put on the arm of the person to be vaccinated and a small scratch made so that the live organism can enter the skin. The resulting sore spot heals quickly and usually causes little, if any, upset.

Routine childhood vaccination against smallpox has now been discontinued. In future, only children going into areas where smallpox is prevalent will require vaccination, but it is important that such children should be re-vaccinated every three years.

Vaccination should not be carried out if any member of the family has eczema. Women should not be vaccinated at any time during pregnancy unless there has been direct contact with a smallpox patient. An injection of a substance called gamma globulin is then given at the same time. Vaccination should be postponed if the person has been in contact with someone with an infectious disease, a boil, or an infected wound.

When weakened germs are given to a person he will contract a mild illness which, in turn, will develop antibodies to protect him against a severe form of that illness in the future. This 'immunization' can last for years. Also an altered toxin can be injected to provoke the production of antibodies. Diphtheria, whooping cough (pertussis), and lockjaw (tetanus) can be prevented in this way, and these three vaccinations are usually given in a single injection called 'triple vaccine'. Three injections of this triple vaccine are given during the baby's first year, followed by a booster dose of diphtheria and tetanus vaccine at the age of five years.

Poliomyelitis vaccine is given by injection, or by mouth, (usually on a lump of sugar) in three doses during the first year of life. Vaccine should not be given by mouth if diarrhoea is present.

Measles vaccine is given at about fifteen months and protection against tuberculosis (by BCG) in the early 'teens. (School authorities now test all children between the ages of ten to thirteen to determine whether they are immune to tuberculosis. Those who are negative reactors are given the BCG.) Travellers to certain countries are advised to have immunizing injections against typhoid and paratyphoid fevers and a booster dose of polio vaccine. This should be given two–three months before departure, if possible. In

1973 the World Health Organization declared that immunization against cholera is no longer necessary unless an epidemic is prevalent. Some countries, however, insist on all immigrants holding a certificate of cholera immunization. Details may be obtained from the appropriate Embassy.

Oral poliomyelitis, BCG, and smallpox vaccines should not be given to persons receiving cortisone treatment or recovering from an illness.

All records of immunization should be kept carefully.

Most young girls now receive vaccination against German measles. It is possible that a pregnant woman who contracts German measles during the first three months of pregnancy may give birth to an abnormal baby, but this is not always so.

The following table sets out the usual ages at which immunization is given:

Age	Immunization
4–6 months	Diphtheria/Tetanus/Pertussis vaccine Poliomyelitis vaccine (oral)
6–8 months	Diphtheria/Tetanus/Pertussis vaccine Poliomyelitis vaccine (oral)
12–14 months	Diphtheria/Tetanus/Pertussis vaccine Poliomyelitis vaccine (oral)
15–24 months	Measles vaccine
5 years (or at school entry)	Diphtheria/Tetanus vaccine Poliomyelitis vaccine (oral)
10–13 years	BCG
11–13 years (girls)	Rubella (German measles)
School leavers	Poliomyelitis vaccine Tetanus vaccine

Some infectious diseases

Measles

The incubation period is ten to fourteen days.

At the end of this time the patient appears to have a cold with a running nose, slight cough, red eyes and a fever. Small white patches, called koplik spots, appear on the lining of the mouth.

After a further three to nine days a red blotchy rash appears behind the ears and the forehead and then, over the next day or two, covers the face and body. It fades slowly over a period of about one week.

A certain amount of bronchitis is present in every case of measles, but antibiotics are not necessary unless pneumonia or an inflamed ear (see Chapter 8) develops. If croup (noisy, distressed breathing) develops, medical advice should be sought immediately. If the child dislikes a bright light, it may be soothing to him to have the room darkened.

Whooping cough (Pertussis)

The incubation period is six to eighteen days.

The onset of this disease is gradual.

After this time the patient appears to have a severe head cold and (sometimes) bronchitis.

During the following seven days the cough becomes severe, especially at night, and then the paroxysmal stage develops: the child makes twenty to thirty *short* coughs and then draws in breaths, producing the characteristic 'whooping' noise. Vomiting sometimes occurs.

This stage lasts for two weeks or more, the 'whoops' becoming less frequent.

A slight cough will persist for several months afterwards, and the tendency to 'whoop' may recur when the child catches subsequent colds. This does not mean that he has a second attack of whooping cough, merely that he has established a habit of 'whooping', but this will disappear in time. It is wise to prevent irritants such as a smoke-filled room, or a sudden change in temperature.

Side effects of attacks

Some children develop bleeding of the eye (i.e. rupture of the small blood vessels in the eye) during a severe attack of coughing. Although this looks alarming it is not dangerous and will not affect the sight.

Small ruptures (of the abdominal muscles) can also occur but usually these right themselves during convalescence.

131

Some dangers of whooping cough

Whooping cough can be a serious and even deadly infection in children under one year old, because of the possibility of pneumonia developing. Young babies should not be exposed to this disease.

Some children do not develop the characteristic 'whoop' but, instead, have spasms of 'breath-holding' which can be very alarming and dangerous. Skilled nursing care is necessary and admission to hospital may be arranged.

Lasting damage to the lungs can be prevented by active treatment, and medical advice should always be sought.

Children who are sick frequently during attacks lose weight and become more prone to complications. They should be re-fed after being sick and small, frequent meals given.

Mumps

The incubation period is seventeen to twenty-one days.

The onset is fairly sudden with a painful swelling of the face due to swollen salivary glands. This may occur on one or both sides.

There is a loss of appetite.

This stage of the illness may last anything from a few days to a week.

Mumps usually is a mild disease but it may be accompanied by meningitis, or it may take the form of meningitis without the swelling of the face.

In an adult female there is sometimes painful swelling of the breasts; and, in the male, of the testicles. Children may develop stomach pains and sickness. This is not dangerous and usually clears up of its own accord. No vaccine is available against this disease.

Chicken pox

The incubation period is eleven to twenty-one days (the average is about eighteen days).

In healthy children it is usually a mild disease.

The first signs are crops of small red spots on the chest and abdomen. These become blisters and may scab. Care must be taken to avoid scratching or pock marks may remain.

There is a general 'unwell feeling' for approximately ten days.

Chicken pox may occur after contact with someone with 'shingles' (herpes zoster); less frequently, shingles develops as a result of contact with chicken pox. No vaccine is available.

German measles (rubella)

The incubation period is fourteen to twenty-one days.

It is usually a mild illness with a slight fever at the onset.

The small glands in the neck are usually enlarged. The rash of small pink spots lasts for a few days only and is less blotchy than that of measles. The disease can be caught only once in a lifetime but many other slight infections cause a similar rash and may be taken for recurrent attacks of German measles.

Glandular fever

The cause of this illness is uncertain but it appears to be spread by close personal contact, such as kissing.

The disease has three forms – anginose, febrile and glandular.

The incubation period is fourteen to twenty one days.

The anginose form. This is the commonest form, especially in young adults. The patient has a sore throat, the neck glands are very swollen (obviously so), and breathing and swallowing may be difficult. The glands in the armpits and groins may be slightly enlarged. The patient runs a temperature of 37·2°C to 37·8°C. The membrane at the back of the throat is white and remains so for a week or more.

The febrile form. In this form there are no definite symptoms other than fever and a general feeling of being unwell.

The glandular form. This form is common in young children. There is fever, and the glands in the armpits, the neck and groins are swollen.

Diagnosis of this disease can be confirmed by blood tests. It is not a serious disease and most patients recover in two to three weeks.

Treatment:

The main treatment is to give plenty of fluids. A kaolin poultice on the painful glands may be comforting (see page 76).

There is no vaccine available against glandular fever.

Scarlet Fever

The incubation period is one to three days.

A sore throat, due to an infection called streptococcal, is a common condition but a more serious type of infection causes painful red tonsils with a fever and, sometimes, sickness. The tongue is usually coated.

The infection can spread to the ear (see Chapter 8), or produce a poison or toxin causing 'scarlet fever'. The latter is characterized by a scarlet rash, which appears the day after the onset of the illness and covers the whole body. The face appears flushed while the area around the mouth is whiter than usual.

As the rash fades the skin peels. This skin is not infectious.

In recent years streptococcal infections such as scarlet fever have become less severe as antibiotics are usually prescribed by the doctor.

Admission to hospital is not necessary unless a complication affecting the kidneys or heart develops, but nowadays, because the illness is 'nipped in the bud', this rarely happens.

To prevent the spread of infection it is important to see that children with running noses or ears use paper handkerchiefs and that these are burnt after use.

Typhoid and paratyphoid fevers

Now that more people are holidaying abroad every year there has been an increase in the number of cases of typhoid and paratyphoid in this country. Acute meningitis sometimes develops and the results may be fatal.

The early symptoms of these fevers may be vague, with headache, fever, loss of appetite and constipation. Symptoms do not develop until two or three weeks after swallowing the organism.

In many foreign countries notices can be seen advising against drinking tap water. This advice should be taken, and applied, not only when staying in the countryside or remote villages, but also in some of the big towns. Salads, ices and ice cubes should also be avoided.

Medical advice must be sought if any of the above symptoms develop after returning from a holiday abroad.

Unfortunately, people who have caught the infection may continue to 'carry' it for some time after they recover. Personal hygiene, especially with regard to the handling of food, and thorough washing of the hands under running water, is important at all times.

Acute meningitis (inflammation of the meninges of the brain and spinal cord).

This disease usually begins very suddenly with sickness and acute pain in the head and neck. Later, a rash develops. Immediate admission to hospital is essential.

Lockjaw (Tetanus)

This is a serious condition characterized by spasms in the muscles following the infection of cuts, grazes and scratches.

The muscles of the face are the first to be affected, resulting in twisting of the mouth and 'grimacing'.

Admission to hospital is essential.

Immunization against tetanus can be combined with diphtheria and whooping cough immunizations or, in the case of adults, given separately.

Infantile paralysis (acute poliomyelitis)

The campaign in the UK for immunization of children against poliomyelitis has been very successful and the disease is now rare in this country.

135

The vaccine can be given by injection or in the form of drops on a lump of sugar.

During an epidemic, infection is often widespread but comparatively few victims develop paralysis.

The disease may appear as a mild illness with fever, headache and general aching as in influenza (see Chapter 8), or it may take the form of tonsilitis with some glands of the neck becoming swollen. It has also been known to begin with loose stools and sickness. Paralysis is often brought about by fatigue or injury during the early stages, and for this reason, absolute rest is essential during the days when the illness is at the acute stage.

If the muscles of the legs or arms appear weak, the doctor should be informed without delay.

In the presence of an epidemic, full precautions must be taken to isolate the patient and barrier nursing must be practised whilst awaiting admission to hospital.

11. Nursing a patient with a skin disease

Some general points

A skin disease may arise from a cause outside, or inside, the patient. Many are inherited. Mental stress and psychological upsets influence skin diseases, but only rarely are they the primary cause.

The agents may be irradiation (i.e. severe sunburn), an irritant (i.e. detergent) or a living organism, such as a virus or a mite (scabies).

Systemic diseases such as diabetes mellitus or malignant disease can make the skin more liable to infection by bacteria, yeasts and fungi.

Itching is the most common symptom of skin disease and can range from being just uncomfortable to being distressing and unbearable. It is helpful to keep the room cool.

Sedatives for day as well as night time are often prescribed as also are antihistamine drugs. Absolute rest in bed is not often necessary, but when the patient is in bed, he should not lie on rubber or plastic undersheets as these will only aggravate the condition. Incontinent pads should be used if there is any danger of soiling the bed linen.

Because skin conditions cause mental and physical discomfort it is necessary to reassure the patient. On no account must he be made to feel unclean. If his skin disease is contagious, it is wise to take all precautions, but he must not receive the impression that you are afraid to go near him. If care is taken he can be nursed and handled as competently as any other patient.

Baths

Baths are usually comforting if they are allowed, as they help to remove previous applications of creams and ointments, as well as skin crusts and scales. The water should be warm, not hot, and the patient should stay in the bath no longer than five minutes. He should not 'towel' himself but gently pat himself dry.

The cream/paint/lotion which has been prescribed by his doctor should be applied immediately after the bath.

Emulsifying ointment baths may be given to people with a chronic dry eczema, where dryness of the skin is troublesome. The emulsifying ointment, prescribed by the doctor, is dissolved in a small quantity of very hot water and mixed well with the bath water. A less greasy solution such as aqueous cream BNF is sometimes prescribed. This is often very soothing. Again, mix the cream well into a little very hot water first to prevent it 'lumping' or 'floating'.

Potassium permanganate baths may be ordered for some infections. The correct strength can be obtained by adding 60 ml of potassium permanganate solution 1:8.000 to an ordinary size bath of warm water. If crystals are used, great care must be taken to see that they are thoroughly and completely dissolved as they can cause small burns if they are allowed to come into direct contact with the skin.

Coal-tar baths are usually ordered in the treatment of psoriasis. If 60 ml of coal tar solution is added to a bath of warm water, loose scales over the affected areas can be very, very, gently removed.

Ointments and creams

The advent of corticosteroid preparations has revolutionized the treatment of many skin diseases, especially those of the eczema group. The usual preparations prescribed are Synalar and Betnovate. Usually a 1 in 4 dilution is ordered. Sometimes an antiseptic is added to the cream to treat or prevent infection. Coal-tar ointments and antifungal creams are also available.

Application

Put on a disposable polythene glove and apply a thin layer of the prescribed cream to the affected area. Rub in very gently – but well. Do not use cotton wool or gauze for the application as the gentle rubbing is an essential part of treatment.

It is important to report any change in the skin condition to the family doctor on his next visit.

Dressings

Stockinette gauze makes an excellent covering: it is quickly applied, comfortable, and allows air to circulate freely. Sometimes cortisone creams have to be covered by polythene to provide an air-tight covering. This aids preservation of the ointment or cream and keeps in moisture. Polythene bags can be used for hands and feet: sheeting is necessary for arms, legs and body, but this covering is usually ordered for night time only.

Polythene or plastic bags and sheeting should not be used for small children as there is the danger of the child removing them and suffocating if they pull them over the face.

Bandages

Several types of impregnated bandages are available and can be used for wrapping when a whole limb is affected. The medicament contained in the bandage is usually ichthyol, used for varicose ulcers, coal tar, or a corticosteroid. It is important not to bandage too tightly as this can cause the patient much discomfort.

If a supportive bandage is ordered, a stout elastic one is more effective than a crêpe one. The bandage should extend from the toes to the knee or even further up the thigh. If the foot is not included, any tendency to the collection of fluid in the tissues is likely to be made worse.

Viral infections

Warts

The common wart is caused by a virus.
Warts are frequently found on the hands, and on the soles of children's feet. They are contagious: that is, they can be spread by touch. Although various destructive techniques can be used in an attempt to clear them, they will eventually disappear of their own accord.

Cold sore (herpes simplex)

This is the common cold sore which often breaks out on the lips. The virus is present in the body and responds to a stimulus such as fever, sunburn, or an illness such as pneumonia. These sores usually resolve spontaneously when the cause is dealt with and the body's defences are built up again.

Shingles (herpes zoster)

This disease is also caused by a virus. It tends to occur in older people who have had chicken pox in childhood. What stimulates the virus again is not known. A rash breaks out and there is pain – often severe and persistent. The rash has a red base with very fine blisters on top, and it creeps round the body along the route of a nerve (herpes = creeping and zoster = girdle). The most common sites are the waist, chest and forehead. Codein or Anadin may help in the relief of pain, but stronger analgesics may be necessary and, if so,

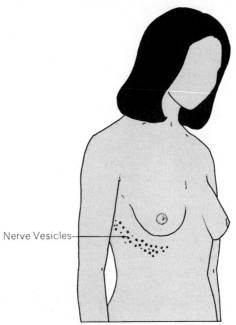

Nerve Vesicles

Shingles: the rash follows the line of the nerve

140

will be prescribed by the doctor. The affected area should be kept dry. The main task when looking after someone who has shingles is to keep up his morale because the pain lasts a long time and is very severe. This is especially so in older people. It is also debilitating and convalescence may be slow.

Bacterial infections

Some bacteria cause skin diseases. A septic spot is an infection of a hair root: a pus-filled nodule, which sometimes develops, is called a boil or furuncle. Boils are more common in hairy areas such as the armpit and at the back of the neck.

If a series of boils appears, medical advice should be sought, as this can indicate general 'run-down-ness' or even the beginning of diabetes mellitus (sugar diabetes).

Infection just under the skin can be impetigo. This takes the form of inflamed weepy patches with yellow crusts. It often begins on the face. Impetigo occurs mostly in school-children and is highly contagious. A high standard of personal hygiene should be observed and all towels, flannels, handkerchiefs, etc., kept separate from those belonging to other members of the family.

Small septic spots can be healed by the application of an anti-bacterial paint or cream. A crop of boils may require a course of antibiotics, whilst impetigo is usually treated with an antibiotic ointment. All these must be prescribed by a doctor.

Absolute and scrupulous cleanliness is essential when caring for people with these infections.

Yeast infections

Monilia is the commonest yeast infection. It appears as 'thrush' in babies' mouths and as white patches on the vulva of some diabetic and pregnant women.

It may cause patches of inflammation between folds of the skin in very fat people (under the breast or in the groin). It can be treated with a paint such as gentian violet, or with a cream such as Vioform or Nystatin.

These may be prescribed by the doctor. Again, close attention to personal hygiene and scrupulous cleanliness is an essential part of the treatment.

Fungal infections

Some pathogenic fungi feed and multiply in the horny layer of the skin, in the hair, and on the nails.

Fungus of the scalp hair causes scaling bald patches in school children.

Fungus of the body skin can be caught from animals. The lesions are round, hence the name 'ringworm'. Chronic forms occur in the groins, nails and between the toes.

Griseofulvin is effective against most varieties of fungus. It is an antibiotic and can only be prescribed by a doctor.

Skin ringworm can be treated by the application of Whitefield's ointment (compound benzoic acid) but an antibiotic taken by mouth is usually necessary for scalp and nail ringworm.

Terminology of skin lesions

Macule — a flat spot of a different colour from the surrounding skin, e.g. freckle.

Papule — a small lump raised above the skin surface.

Nodule — a more deeply attached lump.

Scale — a flat collection of shed horny cells.

Crust — a dried deposit – usually serum – on the skin.

Blister — a skin bleb filled with a clear fluid.

Vesicle — a very small blister.

Pustule — a skin bleb filled with pus.

Excoriation — damage to the skin – scratchings and superficial cuts.

Cyst — a fluid filled cavity.

Erythema — redness of the skin.

Erosion — superficial loss of skin.

Ulcer — an area with loss of full thickness of skin (in gastric ulcer the term applies to mucous membrane.)

Athlete's foot

This is usually, but not always, a fungus infection and is a form of ringworm. It appears as pink peeling patches between and under the toes. It is highly contagious.

There are many powders and creams available for this

condition which may be obtained from a chemist. If the condition is not due to a fungus, careful drying and the application of talcum powder will usually suffice.

Baths, bathmats and swimming pools are well known as sources of infection and it is for this reason that it is unwise to walk in bare feet around public pools and baths.

In hotels, etc., care should be taken when using bathmats, especially those made of cork.

It is important to dry the feet very well after bathing, especially between and under the toes. Socks, stockings and shoes should be considered infected and changed and washed carefully.

Scabies

This is a skin disease caused by a minute parasite or insect which burrows under the skin. The female lays twenty to thirty eggs in the burrow. The eggs hatch out in seven days and the young then burrow out in different directions. In four weeks they become adult. The males die after mating and the females are left to lay their eggs and restart the cycle. The females can usually be found in the white spot at the end of each burrow. The commonest sites of infection are the hands (especially between the fingers) the tummy, and the feet. The irritation is worse when the skin becomes warm – i.e. at night time.

There are many cleaning services available for these patients. Here they are given a hot bath and a special lotion such as benzyl benzoate or gamma benzene hexachloride is applied all over the body, omitting the face and neck. The lotion is allowed to dry before clothes are put on.

After twenty-four hours the process is repeated. Twenty-four hours later it is repeated again.

On the fourth day the patient baths and puts on a complete set of clean clothes.

The treatment is repeated one week later, if necessary.

All members of the family sharing the bedroom of the infected person must also be treated, and some authorities treat all members of the patient's family.

The treatment can be given at home if the mother is confident, knowledgeable and conscientious.

12. Nursing a patient with a medical condition

All illnesses not treated by surgery fall into this category. The list is formidable. Only the more common areas can be covered, and those only briefly.

Because many conditions develop with age, some background knowledge of the ageing process may be useful. It is a complex process, and one which is demonstrated in many ways. One of the most 'obvious' ways biologically occurs in the arteries. Very early in life a pathological change begins in the wall of the larger arteries. Fatty material is deposited – in patches at first and more generally later – in and under the smooth linings of these vessels. These gradually 'silt' up, losing their elasticity (atherosclerosis). Sometimes the silting is abrupt and a coronary thrombosis occurs – i.e. an artery in the heart becomes blocked. At other times a cerebral thrombosis occurs – i.e. an artery in the brain becomes blocked. This is sometimes called a 'stroke'. Atherosclerosis is thought to be aggravated by diabetes, hypertension, obesity and cigarette smoking. It is uncommon in women before the menopause.

Blood carried by arteries is vital to individual cells. It brings fuel and oxygen with it so that the fuel can be burnt to supply the energy necessary to enable cells to survive and to work; it carries raw materials to secretory cells, thus enabling them to produce their secretions; and it carries hormones which activate function.

Gradual deprivation of blood supply to cells results in failure of tissues to replace themselves adequately.

Signs of old age

Physical

The hair loses its colour, changes texture, becomes thin and disappears.

The skin changes in texture, appearance and colour.

Muscle tone is less and movement becomes slower.
There is degeneration of the bone and stooping occurs.
The senses of sight, hearing, taste and smell are less acute.
The appetite becomes smaller.
The teeth decay/fall out.
The pattern of sleep alters from the normal individual pattern built up over the years.

Psychological

The mental processes slow down: e.g. it takes longer to learn a new skill (important to remember, this, when rehabilitating a 'stroke patient').
New ideas are less acceptable.
There is less inclination to experiment or take risks.
Recollections of recent events are poor whilst memories, sayings and experiences of earlier days come clearly to mind.

Prevention of illness in the elderly

Not everyone looks forward eagerly to retirement; although anticipated, it can often be a very unhappy experience when it actually happens.

Some employers, local authorities and voluntary organizers now run courses designed to 'educate' people in how best to use their increased leisure hours and enjoy a useful and happy retirement.

A certain amount of degeneration after retirement age is inevitable, but many conditions can be prevented if the first signs are recognized and treated.

Some local authorities have established clinics for the 'over sixty-fives' where routine medical examinations are carried out, and advice given.

A complete cure may be effected if signs and symptoms of disease are recognized and treated in the early stages. If a disease is allowed to advance, it may be possible only to alleviate the suffering.

Much illness of old age could be prevented if a balanced diet is adhered to. Those who live alone especially do not feed themselves well and their diet is often insufficient in force as well as quantity. Plenty of proteins and fresh fruit should be eaten, and two litres of fluid should be drunk every day.

It is important to keep the home warm. The temperature of the living room, and the bedroom, should be not less than 16°C. Old people, as well as babies, can suffer from hypothermia (see Chapter 19).

Physical illness cannot be considered in isolation and in old people emotional and mental disturbance can be great. There is also the fear of loss of independence – and of death.

Worry and anxiety can often be relieved by the judicial use of drugs: sedation may be necessary at night but not until other treatment has been tried. The giving of drugs should be supervised as old people are often forgetful and a double dose may be taken inadvertently.

It is important always to remember that elderly people have, like everyone else, dignity and self respect.

They are sensitive to atmosphere and attitudes: they must be made to feel not only wanted but needed.

In strange surroundings they may experience fear and anxiety. Often they are afraid of being thought a nuisance and therefore are shy and hesitant about expressing a need, a desire, or a worry.

Their reactions are slower; they may find it difficult to answer a question; speech may become slurred, slow, repetitive.

Patience is the keynote when you are with old people. Often their companionship is a privilege and their conversation wise and entertaining.

It is difficult to define an 'elderly' person. Some people are active and energetic in their nineties; others are slow and disinclined to take risks in their fifties.

The main aim in the management of health and illness is to preserve the function of all faculties – the most important being the mental functions for, when these deteriorate, the consequences can be disastrous. Work, study, reading, day or evening classes, theatres, conversation, hobbies – activities such as these are vital if mental alertness is to be maintained.

When an elderly person is ill, many members of the curing and caring professions may be needed, for it is then that all supporting services should be made available: not only are there doctors and nurses to help, but also physiotherapists, occupational therapists, chiropodists, health visitors and social workers. To advise on equipment, bedding and to provide auxiliary nursing help to relieve you, there are the local Red Cross and St John Ambulance, the WRVS, the Old People's Welfare Association, mobile libraries, meals-on-wheels, and other organizations.

If you don't know what help is available in your area, contact the local Voluntary Aid Service (Red Cross or St John) or the Citizens' Advice Bureau, who will have lists of services such as clubs, day centres, remedial exercise classes, laundry services, etc.

If adaptations or fittings are needed in a house to accommodate an old person or to make life easier for him or her, the Social Services department should be contacted. The health visitor or doctor will tell you how to do this.

The dangers of bedfastness

Bedfastness of the elderly is to be avoided. If acutely ill, obviously a period in bed is necessary, but bedfastness over a period of time renders the elderly vulnerable. Bodily functions deteriorate and complications set in.

Diseases of old age are almost always multiple. When one manifests itself others will often be diagnosed at the same time. Often 'the multiple deficiency syndrome' is present – i.e. malnutrition, anaemia, deficiency of hormones, thyroid, blood supply, arterial function, and so on. Hypertension, arthritis, defective teeth, lack of vision, bad hearing, painful feet, etc., are common. There may be obesity, diabetes, infection of the lungs or urinary tract.

Eyes should be tested regularly: there should be regular visits to the dentist and chiropodist; and a hearing aid provided, if necessary.

When an old person is kept in bed there is danger of:
1. Muscles becoming weak and flabby.
2. Bones becoming thin (and therefore prone to breaking).
3. Joints stiffening and contractions appearing.
4. Foot drop.

5. Deterioration and weakness of bladder and bowel, often resulting in complete lack of control.
6. Constipation (sometimes with impaction of faeces).
7. Loss of appetite.
8. Pressure sores.
9. Hypostatic pneumonia.
10. Venous stagnation, leading to thrombosis and embolism.

Lost body functions are difficult to regain and all old people must be safeguarded against inactivity. In all illnesses it is important to get the patient moving as soon as possible but it is especially important when the patient is elderly.

It should be stressed here that the exercising of all joints through the whole range of movement twice a day is of the utmost importance. Ask the physiotherapist or nurse to show you how to do 'passive movements'. Every effort and improvement made should be praised and encouraged. Certain procedures, such as dressing, walking to the lavatory, and joining the family for meals, should be undertaken by the patient as soon as possible.

Nutrition

As age increases the body cells change and the basic metabolic rate falls.

As a result, the body requires less food. But the food that is eaten must have a high nutritional content. Protein is important. Meat, fish, cheese or eggs should be eaten at least once a day. Careful cooking is essential to tempt a capricious appetite and to ensure that all nutrients are contained. Protein does not have to be the expensive kind; liver, herrings and sardines are rich in fat and vitamin D, as well as in protein.

Milk contains all nutrients and half a pint a day is the minimum an old person should have. If fruit and vegetables are not taken in sufficient quantities, Bemax may be added to the breakfast cereal or porridge.

Small, frequent, attractively served meals are very important for the elderly sick person.

Arterial disease

There are several types of chronic obliterative disease from which the elderly may suffer:

1. Atherosclerosis (a degenerative condition of the artery walls).
2. Embolism or thrombosis (a clot of blood forming).
3. Venous thrombosis (a clot of blood in a vein, usually affecting the lower limbs).

Medical treatment is necessary for all, and the physician's instructions must be carried out implicitly.

Overall nursing care must be given.

Strokes (cerebro-vascular accidents)

'Strokes' are due to haemorrhage, thrombosis or embolus in the brain (cerebrum).

Cerebral haemorrhage is caused by the rupture of an artery or aneurysm in the brain and occurs in patients with high blood pressure. It cuts off the blood supply to the affected part of the brain and sometimes leaking blood also causes pressure on adjacent areas.

The onset is abrupt, with a headache, mental confusion and paralysis of one side of the body. Sometimes the patient loses consciousness very quickly.

Cerebral thrombosis is due to the clotting of blood in an artery of the brain, usually as the result of atherosclerosis (a form of arteriosclerosis, in which there is fatty degeneration of the middle coat of the arterial walls). The effect of this depends on the size and importance of the blood vessel concerned, and varies from slight weakness in one limb to paralysis of one side of the body, or even coma.

If the thrombosis extends, anticoagulants (drugs to prevent clotting of the blood) are given. General nursing care is necessary.

Cerebral embolism is due to obstruction of an artery in the brain by a clot formed either in the heart or on a patch of atheroma in a carotid artery (the large neck blood vessel).

Treatment is aimed at preventing further attacks.

It is as well to remember that the disability from a stroke is at its greatest during the first few days; improvement is continuous but slow from that time for two to three months. Any disability remaining after two to three months is likely to become permanent, but this depends on the severity of the stroke and the age of the patient.

If a person survives a stroke for forty-eight hours, his chances of recovery (even if not to a full extent) are high.

The immediate treatment for stroke patients is given in hospitals, but general nursing care may be needed for some time after discharge.

Again, it is important to encourage ambulation and activity.

Physiotherapy should be continued. Help may be needed in dressing, feeding, washing and getting to the lavatory.

Communication may be difficult. If speech is totally absent, you may find yourself your patient's mouthpiece and interpreter. But even if he is unable to speak, his treatment, its purpose, the anticipated result and the value of his collaboration must be explained to him. Although a patient may be unable to speak after a stroke he can hear, and it is important to remember that *hearing is the first sense to return after a period of unconsciousness and the last to leave before unsconsciousness sets in*. In fact, treat your patient like a normal human being – after all, that's what he is!

It is rewarding to establish a sign language – a nod, a wink, a lifting of the eyebrows, etc. Keep a pad and pencil handy if the patient is able to write, but anticipation of his needs will be even more appreciated. Try to put yourself in your patient's place and understand his wishes.

Rehabilitation after a heart attack

A heart attack is caused by hardening of the arteries supplying the heart muscles with blood, and the pain and tightness experienced during an attack is comparable to the cramp which develops in the calf muscles of long-distance runners and footballers. Both develop because too great a demand is

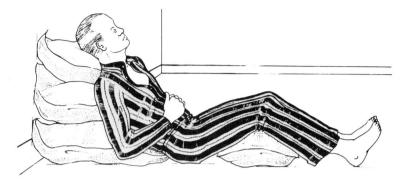

Recumbent position for nursing a patient after a heart attack

made on the muscle. Given the right conditions the muscle recovers its normal strength and functions effectively.

The duration of rest in bed will be determined by the extent of the impact and by the clinical condition of the patient.

One of the best and least expensive 'heart beds' is a traditional armchair. Using a commode requires less effort than balancing on a bedpan. The majority of these patients cared for at home can use both the commode and chair for short periods forty-eight hours after the attack. Some family doctors get their patients sitting in a chair for several hours a day by the tenth day; others advise three weeks of bed rest, with only short periods out of bed. Your own doctor and nurse will give you individual advice.

Most would agree that each patient requires individual assessment, but generally, the older the patient, the shorter the period of bed rest.

Four weeks after suffering an attack, the majority of patients are dressed and taking light exercise. Most need a further six to eight weeks off work. After that time, the family doctor should be consulted regarding the future way of life.

Many patients are able to resume their work and hobbies provided these do not involve heavy manual labour or lifting heavy weights. Some may need to seek premature retirement or be referred to the Rehabilitation Officer for assessment.

Driving a car imposes considerable stress and is best avoided for at least two months after an attack. Lorry and bus drivers may have to change their occupations.

Regular exercise, particularly walking, should be encouraged, and the patient should live as full a life as possible
Conditions likely to bring on an attack are:

1. Prolonged effort, such as walking too fast, or uphill, or lifting a heavy weight.
2. A full stomach (small meals are the answer).
3. Sudden change of temperature.
4. Emotion – tension, frustration (such as being stuck in a traffic jam).

It is important that the patient understands that pain is a warning signal which should be heeded.

If pain is felt, the person concerned should stop and wait. Anticipation of pain is useful. Encourage your patient to judge for himself how best to minimize the pain by avoiding over-taxation. He should avoid all situations which make him tense and give himself extra time to catch buses and trains.

Diet

Small meals should be taken, and foods which produce flatulence avoided. Butter, milk, cream, cheese and the fat of meat should be restricted, as should starch and sugar.

Alcohol, tea and coffee in moderation are not harmful.

Sleep

Adequate, relaxed sleep is important. If this is difficult, the family doctor should be consulted regarding sedation at night. If possible, encourage your patient to empty his mind of all worrying thoughts before going to bed. Stress and strain in all forms should be avoided.

Smoking

Cigarettes should not be smoked. Some physicians allow an occasional pipe or cigar.

Finally, remember that this is a condition which is compatible with a very full and useful life. With common sense and treatment it may improve quite dramatically!

ICI have produced a worthwhile booklet, *Living with your Heart*, which can be obtained direct from them (Imperial Chemical Industries Ltd, Imperial Chemical House, Millbank, SW1).

Hiatus hernia

When a portion of the stomach moves upwards through the hole in the diaphragm and into the chest, this is called an oesophago-gastric hernia. It is a fairly common condition which occurs in older or fat people, and may be without symptoms. When these do occur there is acid regurgitation into the mouth, heartburn, and a burning sensation behind the breast bone. These conditions are made worse by tight corsets, bending forward, and obesity.

Treatment consists of reduction of weight (see page 60 for diet), the administration of antacids (magnesium trisilicate BP, milk of magnesia, etc.), and avoidance of the aggravating factors. If the symptoms are troublesome at night the head of the bed should be raised on blocks (safety and stability must be ensured) and the pillows arranged to prevent the patient slipping down in the bed.

If the symptoms are not relieved, or if iron deficiency or ulceration occurs, surgery may be considered.

Peptic ulcers

A peptic ulcer is caused by acid-digestion of the mucosa of the stomach. It can be a gastric ulcer or a duodenal ulcer.

There is a tendency for gastric and duodenal ulcers to run in families. Both cause pain, radiating through to the back, often worse *before* meals and briefly relieved *by* meals. In the early stages the pain may be relieved by milk, and antacids. Vomiting may also relieve the pain. Heartburn, nausea and loss of weight are common.

It is usually best to eat little and often. The food which aggravates the condition – usually fried, spiced, curried and pickled foods – should be noted and avoided. To reduce acid secreted by the stomach, antacids may be given (magnesium trisilicate, aluminium hydroxide or calcium carbonate are recommended). The family doctor may prescribe medicines. If so, these should be given punctually (see page 66). Rest is helpful and if this is impossible at home, admission to hospital is sometimes arranged.

'Slipped disc' (prolapsed intervertebral disc)

This is probably one of the most common diagnoses of our time and may occur as a result of a strain or injury. It is the commonest cause of low back pain when a disc in the lumbar spine is affected.

A prolapse may also occur in the cervical or dorsal areas.

There is pain, weakness of legs or arms (depending on which disc is affected), tingling and numbness in the hands, fingers or feet, inability to stand erect or to walk without listing to one side. Home treatment consists of rest in bed with a board under a thin hair or Dunlopillo mattress.

The aim of rest and support is to provide the opportunity for natural changes to take place in the lesion, i.e. local oedema will subside, thus reducing pressure. Physiotherapy in the form of heat, traction and exercises plays a most important part in the treatment.

Some surgeons advocate a plaster of Paris jacket: additional support may be obtained from a made-to-measure 'surgical belt'.

Rehabilitation should include instruction in the correct ways of lifting, stretching and picking up heavy objects.

Surgery is undertaken only when management along the above lines has proved ineffective.

Parkinson's disease

Parkinson's disease is one of the most common chronic diseases of the nervous system. It is a disorder of the large groups of nerve cells deep in the brain which are responsible for movement. The exact cause is unknown. Both sexes are affected and the onset is usually in middle life.

It is a slowly progressive disorder, characterized by a mask-like face, slowness of voluntary movement, rigidity of muscles and tremor at rest (this usually disappears on movement). There may also be a disturbance of balance, the patient tending to fall backwards or sideways.

The initial treatment is the administration of drugs of which there are several alternatives, but instruction concerning their administration must be followed rigidly.

A substance called L-Dopa is now being used and has produced dramatic results in some patients. It has recently been discovered that a combination of L-Dopa with chemical (peripheral dopa decarboxylase) inhibitors allows a reduction in L-Dopa in dosage, a quicker clinical response and cuts down to a very significant degree any side effects. Unfortunately, Parkinson's disease cannot be cured: control is all that can be offered at present.

Some neurologists advocate a form of surgery called stereotactic surgery, to control the tremor and rigidity. Research into the condition continues.

Patients having radiotherapy or deep X-ray treatment

On discharge from hospital following treatment by radiotherapy, patients are given an appointment to return within a few weeks so that the immediate effects of treatment may be observed. Advice should also be given regarding reactions although skin reactions (redness and burning of the skin) are no longer the troublesome feature they were. However, the care of the skin and the avoidance of water on the skin is of great importance and precise instructions should be obtained.

Nausea and sickness can be other unpleasant side effects and the family doctor will be able to prescribe drugs to combat these symptoms.

Patients will need to be tempted to eat, and those having deep X-ray therapy to the mouth, tongue, or tonsils will require soft bland food. Most patients will be encouraged to drink 2–4 litres per day.

If the patient is continuing treatment as an out-patient, encouragement will probably be needed. Transport can often be arranged through the social workers and will cost nothing.

Sometimes chemotherapy (treatment by drugs) will be combined with radiotherapy (treatment by X-ray), and it will be necessary to receive guidance on the diet and fluid intake of these patients. Some foods (such as cheese) are incompatible with some drugs, and because of water retention in the tissues, drinking may have to be restricted.

During both these forms of treatment frequent blood tests will be taken: these are routine and are necessary to find out that the composition of the blood is not being affected by the treatments.

Pain is sometimes experienced by these patients and pain-killing drugs should be prescribed by the hospital or family doctor. Sedatives or sleeping pills are not enough as they do not kill pain. For sleeping, a pain killer may be given in addition to the sleeping pill.

13. Nursing a patient who has had an operation

People who have been seriously ill or who have undergone major surgery may be transferred from hospital to a special convalescent or recovery home. However, most patients, if they are able, prefer to convalesce in their own home.

Help or advice should be sought from the patient's own doctor. If daily visits from a trained nurse are needed, this can be arranged from the National Health Service, either through the ward sister or social worker before discharge from hospital or, if the patient is already at home, through the general practitioner. When the full-time services of a trained nurse are required, one of the many agencies who act for private nurses should be contacted. This, again, can be organized through the patient's general practitioner or through the hospital staff. Nursing help can also be obtained from a trained auxiliary nurse, and the local Red Cross or St John Ambulance Headquarters should be contacted if help of a simple basic nursing kind only is required or if occasional relief duty will help the family.

For convalescents (or their families) who need help with housework, shopping, etc., a Home Help may be provided if recommended by the family doctor. If you are able to afford it, a small charge will be made for this service. In most areas a meals-on-wheels service, run by either the National Health Service or a voluntary organization such as the Women's Royal Voluntary Service, will provide, for those in need, a hot meal at least twice a week.

Nursing care should always be planned, and a programme of gradual progression and rehabilitation should be drawn up with the help of the patient's doctor and nurse. Daily routine should also be planned. This will depend on the condition of the patient and the patient's wishes – also the availability of additional help. The patient's needs should be anticipated as far as possible and books, newspapers, writing materials, spectacles, a transistor radio, handker-

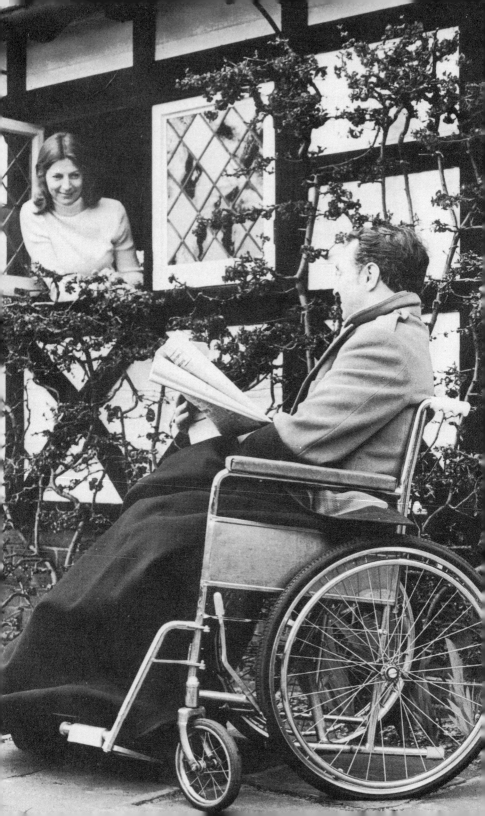

chiefs, and water or fruit juice left within easy reach. Even when the convalescent is ambulant, it is reassuring for him to have a bell to hand, so that he can summon help if necessary. This is particularly important at night. These points can also be applied to medical patients.

Find out when the patient should be given his medicine, how often (and for how long) he is allowed up, how active he may be, and if a special diet is required. It is important also to find out whether fluids should be restricted or if the convalescent should be encouraged to drink.

Advice on how to carry out simple nursing procedures such as bathing, lifting, preventing bedsores (heels and elbows become sore especially quickly in the convalescent patient confined to bed) should be sought from either the nurse, the doctor, or from an auxiliary nurse from one of the Voluntary Aid Societies. If the patient's temperature has to be taken, find out how, how often, when, and how to record it. (see page 35).

It is sometimes difficult to keep the patient's morale high, for convalescence can be a boring time and one resented by a usually active person who wants to return as quickly as possible to normal life. Encouragement is vital at this stage: the patient should be told he is improving and that he looks better. He should be encouraged to pay attention to his appearance. A man may need help with shaving and a woman may need help with her make-up or styling her hair. But always remember that, if the medical attendant permits it, the patient should be allowed to do things for himself as soon as he possibly can.

Rehabilitation to an independent state and to a normal active life should start from the very first day of recovery. Walking aids can be obtained from the local Red Cross Medical Loan depot through the family doctor.

It is always wise to break up the day of a convalescent patient into manageable sessions: boredom and irritability can then be avoided. Organize a fixed routine with set times

When weather conditions permit, the convalescent patient should be encouraged to take short spells in the fresh air and within easy calling distance of those looking after him.

for visitors; put music on before rest-time; arrange activity and exercises after sleep, and so on. In this way, routine becomes reassuring.

Perhaps food is the most important item in a convalescent's day and mealtimes are usually looked forward to eagerly.

If possible, menus should be varied and interesting (the patient's likes and dislikes being taken into consideration).

As soon as he is able, the patient should be helped up for meals and should join the rest of the family in the dining room. When special diets are ordered they must be rigorously adhered to. (For specimen menus see Chapter 5).

Many mothers experience difficulty in feeding a convalescent child. Never ask the child what he would like. The element of surprise is even more important here: too long anticipation blunts a young, capricious, convalescent's appetite. Make mysteries out of meals! Cover the main course with a soup-plate or saucepan lid and remove this with a flourish in front of the invalid. Children also like shapes and patterns so fashion the mashed potatoes into a 'sand castle', cut meat into the squares of a 'staircase', and so on.

Bowel function can be a slight problem during the more inactive stages of convalescence but should never become a major one. Regular habits return when all other functions revert to normal. Never give a laxative without taking professional advice.

When a sick child is convalescing, time should be set aside to play with him or read to him. Help him with any modelling, drawing, or any hobby in which he is interested. It's much more fun playing with someone.

Interesting activities such as collages, jigsaw puzzles, sewing, making felt toys and mobiles, or houses from match boxes, should all be encouraged. To relieve boredom, provide only one toy at a time and remove it before giving another. If a child is surrounded by all his playthings at the same time they will soon all become tedious. Those kept out of sight will be given a warm welcome when produced later on.

Play is possible even when the convalescent child is in bed or lying on a settee. Sew tapes on to a large sheet of waterproof material, pass it round the child's waist, and tie

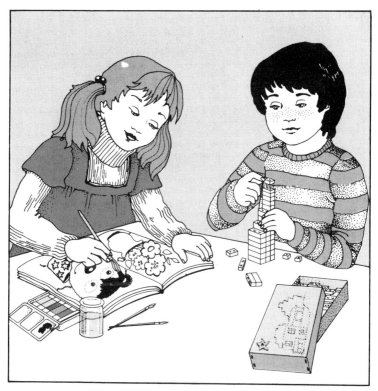

Constructive and creative play

the tapes together under the bed or sofa. He can then paint, model with clay or plasticine to his heart's content.

This kind of sheet also 'collects' lost pieces of jigsaw, sticky paper shapes, pieces of Leggo, small mosaics, building bricks, etc., which all too easily get lost in the bed.

To save your own feet, give the convalescent child a pair of kitchen tongs so that he is able to retrieve for himself anything that falls on the floor. You will find the children's section of the public library usually has books on toymaking, hobbies, and so on. Settling down with a book is a good way of relaxing (not only for the convalescent!) and all sorts of interesting information and knowledge can be gained in this way.

161

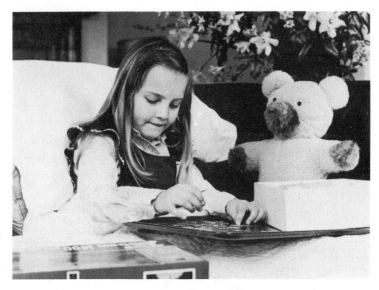

A convalescent child need not be confined to the sickroom, but should have light and airy conditions where she can begin the process of rehabilitation within the family.

Above all, be firm with a convalescent patient: convalescence should be pleasant, but not more enjoyable than normal life! This is especially important with children who may see illness and convalescence as a time when they get their own way and are spoiled. Then begin the problems which arise from children pretending they are ill when, in fact, they are perfectly well. Looking after a convalescent patient can be much more exhausting than caring for an ill one, so keep up your own strength by having regular meals, adequate sleep, and plenty of rest and fresh air.

Special needs after some specific operations

Colostomy

It is sometimes necessary for a patient with a disease of the gut to have part of the gut removed, and for an artificial 'anus' to be made on to the surface of the abdomen. This is called a colostomy. Other people with a disease of the bladder

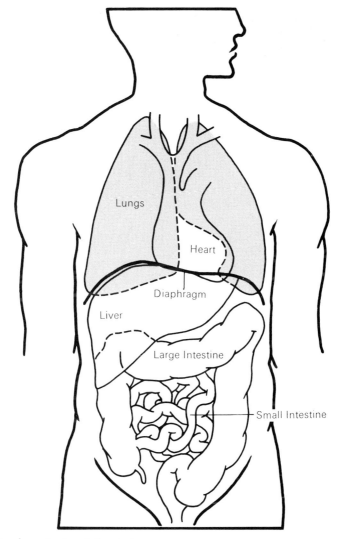

Trunk contents   1 front view

have a short-circuiting operation performed which means that urine is passed through an opening in the abdomen.

This fundamental alteration in the excretion of faeces and urine over which the patient may not have reliable control, can cause strong feelings of shame and humiliation.

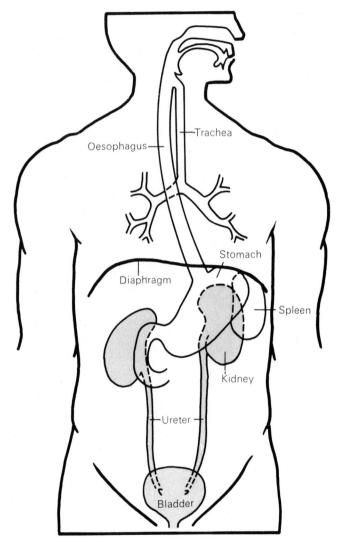

Trunk contents 2 front view

The person concerned may even fear social ostracism and the end of an active and useful life. This is, of course, a totally unnecessarily gloomy view; given encouragement and care, a large proportion of these patients return to their normal jobs and none should suffer socially.

The first essential requirement is sympathetic understanding of the anxiety and the distress, which is a very human reaction to mutilation or abnormality in oneself.

The second is a reliable means of control over excretion by regulation of the bowel or efficient collection of drainage.

The third is the maximum use of the rehabilitation and social services available. The task of rehabilitation is shared between the hospital and the domiciliary staff – and the family. This care begins in the operating theatre where a Stoma Adhesive square to protect the skin and provide a see-through appliance is fitted.

Patients who have an ileostomy (an opening in the part of the gut where the contents are more liquid) or an urinary conduit are fitted with more substantial adherent appliances before leaving hospital. These are usually made of rubber. The patient with a colostomy (an artifical opening into the colon) will continue to use disposable adherent bags. Modern laminated plastic appliances are odour-proof and simple and hygienic to use.

Whatever kind is decided upon, it is essential to see that it is fitted and suited to the patient's needs *before he leaves hospital*. All patients need practice in using their equipment before returning home. Written instructions and advice on diet and general management including the cleaning or disposal of soiled bags should also be collected before discharge.

It is also essential to see that the patient has an adequate supply and knows how to obtain replacements through his own doctor. The name of the appliance and details of its size and type should be given to the family doctor. These patients are entitled to exemption from prescription charges and should complete form EC91, obtainable from any Post Office.

Care of the surrounding skin

Two good non-irritant adhesives now available on prescription are Retina Seal (Davol) and Stoma Adhesive (Squibb). The former is specially suited to patients with an urinary appliance and the latter is most effective on damaged and sore skin.

Skin soreness prevents adhesion of the appliance and allows leakage leading to increased destruction of the surrounding skin. This must be avoided. The causes may include malfunctioning of the stoma (raised opening); an ill-fitting appliance; infection; or the development of an allergy to the appliance material. The advice of the family doctor or nurse should be sought.

A simple treatment which may be ordered is painting the skin with 25 per cent magenta solution and when it is dry, to apply a piece of Stoma Adhesive with a hole cut centrally to accommodate the stoma without constriction. When the adhesive appliance is attached, the dressing should be left in place for a period of up to three days, according to comfort. Applications should continue until the skin is completely healed.

However, the cause of the leakage must be found, and professional help and advice sought immediately.

Views vary concerning the fitting over a colostomy. Some patients feel more secure with an adhesive bag in place all the time; others have actions so certain and regular that they are able to wear gauze dressing and wool over the stoma, held in place by an ordinary roll-on corset.

Many patients find they require to change the flange only once or twice a week.

To clean a colostomy bag, turn it inside out and wash thoroughly with soap and water. Rinse well and leave to drain and dry. If a mild domestic bleach is used to destroy smells, very careful rinsing is necessary.

For some days after the construction of a colostomy, it will act at irregular times. It is important to remember that this will not always be so. Many patients find that they can 'manage' their colostomy as simply as they managed their bowel action. They may, for example, find that action can be induced by drinking a cup of hot tea on wakening. Food has a noticeable effect on a colostomy: for example, onions cause some people to have a loose action. As there is individual variation in the response to food, patients should experiment and keep a notebook, jotting down the foods or drinks which have an adverse effect. Some patients find it useful to thicken the stool by taking cellulose regularly, in the form of Celevac or another proprietary brand. This absorbs water in the gut and swells, producing bulk.

Many associations have built up a useful collection of information and advice on all aspects of stoma care and appliances. These include: the Colostomy Welfare Group, 38–39 Eccleston Square, London SW1V 1PB; the Christie Hospital and Holt Institute, Wilmslow Road, Manchester 20 (tel. no. 061 445 8213); the Ileostomy Association of Great Britain and Ireland, Drove Cottage, Fuzzy Drove, Kempshott, Basingstoke, Hants; the Association for Spina Bifida and Hydrocephalus (ASBAH) National Office, Devonshire Street House, 30 Devonshire Street, London W1N 2EB.

Nursing a patient with a cancerous condition

Cancer is not a disease in itself. It is a generic term covering a wide range of diseases from leukaemia to a mole-like 'spot'. Many of these diseases and conditions have good prognoses but unfortunately 'cancer' has come to mean an implied prognosis of death. This is just not true. Many forms of cancer can be controlled if not cured.

It is important that everyone who comes into contact with these patients has come to terms with the disease themselves. One must have a philosophy so that one is able to be sympathetic without being sentimental, practical without being hard-hearted, and one must be able to impart hope. Lies must be avoided but a prognosis in terms of weeks or months should not be relayed. It is essential to encourage the sick person to live as fully as possible. Patients should not be protected or molly-coddled; they should go out and about, accept social invitations and generally get away from the cushioning life of hospital.

Mastectomy

This means the surgical removal of a breast, and a woman who undergoes this operation has to learn to adapt to the situation. This is not always easy. She will need to be re-assured she will not look different (there are some excellent breast prostheses these days), that she will not be rejected by her husband, fiancé or family and that she will be able to resume sexual relationships.

Fear of looking different is usually great, and most surgeons endeavour to use an incision which will not prevent their patient from wearing low-cut evening dresses. A prosthesis (false breast) is fitted in hospital and usually can be worn as soon as the stitches are removed from the wound.

Often the surgeon or family doctor will talk with the husband or fiancé and the situation can be explained. Also the question of resumption of sexual relationships can be discussed with the appropriate professional adviser. Some advice regarding positions may be necessary but with due sense on both sides and sympathy and understanding on the husband's, this is easily resolved.

Some women experience distaste of their scarred chest. Tact and understanding is required here, together with information and advice on brassières. The district nurse and family doctor will help.

Exercises to keep the arm moving – especially backwards as in dressing the hair – are important and these, together with advice on prostheses and all aspects of rehabilitation, are contained in an excellent leaflet: *Advice to Patients following Mastectomy*, published by the Marie Curie Memorial Foundation. Copies are free, and may be obtained from the Rehabilitation Officer, 124 Sloane Street, London SW1X 9BP. They do ask you to enclose a stamped addressed envelope 6 in × 4 in.

Self-examination of the breast

It is important for all women to know the abnormalities to look for, i.e. a lump, or any change in the shape or size of the breast; if one breast appears slightly larger than the other; any slight pitting (like orange peel), dimpling or puckering – all should be reported to the family doctor. So should any retraction of the nipple or stained discharge from the nipple. It is easy to remember to undertake the self-examination if one does it the same day every month.

Sometimes an operation is necessary to establish the diagnosis. This is particularly so in breast cancer. Not all lumps in the breast are cancerous, but early investigation of any is important. A lump in the breast can be due to mastitis (inflammation of breast tissue), a harmless kind of tumour or cyst, or fatty deposit. Even if the lump is cancerous it can very often be controlled when diagnosed at an early stage. There are thousands of women alive today who had cancer of the breast diagnosed years and years ago. Unfortunately, people who have been cured tend to keep quiet about it.

As disease of the breast is fairly common, it is worth spending a few minutes each month to give yourself a check, for often even the malignant kind can be detected early enough to enable treatment to be carried out, and the disease controlled.

It is a good idea to select a time for regular self-examination, which you are unlikely to forget – e.g., the first day after the end of your period (breasts are usually full and tender immediately before the onset of a period). After the menopause, the first or last day of each month is an obvious time. It is as well to do it at the same time each day, e.g. before going to bed at night or before getting up in the morning.

First, stripped to the waist, stand in a good light in front of a mirror. Look carefully at your reflection for any change or difference in shape, size or colour of breasts or nipples. Also note whether there is any difference in the appearance of the skin and whether it is slightly puckered or dimpled. But, whilst doing this, remember that very few women are symmetrical. Most have one breast higher or larger than the other. What you are looking for is any *recent* change in appearance.

Next, stand with your hands clasped behind your head and see if there is any 'dragging' of one breast. They should both 'lift' in the same way.

For the third stage of the self-examination, lie on your bed without pillows. Place a folded towel under your right shoulder so that it is slightly raised. Put your right hand behind your head. Place your left hand on top of your right breast with the tip of the middle finger just touching the armpit. Feeling with the *flat* of your fingers, draw your hand slowly inwards towards the nipple. Do not use the tips of your fingers, as this will result in 'pinching' or 'clawing' the breast. Lower your hand half an inch at a time and repeat until you have felt all the outer edge of the breast. Do the same over the other half, but this time draw your hand from below upwards, from nipple towards the centre of the breast.

Change the towel to under the left shoulder, place your left hand behind your head and, with your right hand, feel the left breast in the same way.

Normal breast is made of firm tissue with some surface flabbiness and softness. If you detect any alteration in texture, any irregularity or bump or lump, you should consult your doctor at once.

Stained discharge from the nipple should also be reported to your family doctor. (Women who breast feed their babies may find that they continue to express a few drops of milk for several years after feeding has been discontinued. This is clear, and is nothing to worry about).

Head and neck surgery

Sometimes mutilating surgery has to be performed for a cancerous condition of the face, jaw, tongue, mouth, or glands of the neck. In spite of the wonders and excellence of some plastic surgery this mutilation often leads to many problems. Appearance, speech and eating may all be affected and this causes patients to withdraw from social contact and events. This is a great tragedy, for these patients usually have a good prognosis.

Communication difficulties should be helped by a speech therapist in hospital and continued at home. Eating and drinking may require much help – a liquidizer is often a boon. There are many tricks known which enable patients to eat and drink but all need to be adapted to individual patients according to their needs.

Patients need to be encouraged and the family may need help in accepting what may be a difficult situation. Eating can be a messy business and tact and patience will be needed to achieve encouragement and progress.

Neighbours and colleagues at work may also need educating to accept disfigurement and ignore it, for it is vital that these patients are encouraged to live a normal life.

Again the advice of your family doctor and nurse should be sought, whilst the Marie Curie Memorial Foundation will offer invaluable help.

Heart surgery

Congenital heart diseases

These can take many forms and most are now treated by operation. The most common are valve stenoses and septal defects.

1. *Valve stenosis*

Valve cusps do not always develop perfectly, and they may be fused leaving only a very small opening through which the blood is forced. The chamber of the heart near to the

Heart and great vessels

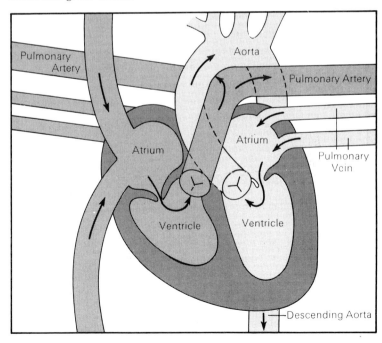

obstructed valve must increase its work to overcome this resistance.

(a) *Pulmonary valve stenosis*
In this condition insufficient blood passes through the pulmonary circulation, causing shortness of breath when exercise is taken. The valve orifice is opened by operation.

(b) *Aortic valve stenosis*
This condition is serious as it affects the main valve from the heart, so the supply of blood to the heart itself as well as that of the systemic circulation, including the brain, is affected. Again, the orifice of the valve may be enlarged by surgery. Sometimes valve replacement is carried out at a later date.

2. *Septal defects*

(a) *Atrial septal defect*
In this condition there is a hole in the septum (muscle wall) between the right and left atria.
   There are four types, all of which are usually treated by surgery.
(b) *Ventricular septal defect*
This also takes the form of a hole in the septum but the hole may be in either the muscular part or the small membraneous part of the wall. Babies with large holes may develop heart failure and surgery is then necessary.
   Some small holes close spontaneously.
   Individual heart surgeons will give advice and instructions regarding their patients upon whom they have performed heart surgery. Descriptions of these operations, which include the insertion of valves and pacemakers are beyond the scope of this book. The after care of these patients must be supervised by the hospital consultant and family doctor and nurse, but it is important that the family receives adequate instructions before the patient is discharged. These must include advice on activity, lifting, drugs, diet (including fluid intake) and attendance at out-patient clinics. The family doctor should be informed immediately the patient returns home.

172

All medicines and drugs must be given at the correct time but this is especially important in the treatment of 'a heart patient'.

Exercise is beneficial but steady relaxed walking rather than hurry is the general rule. Stress and strain should be avoided. Small meals low in fat and sugar should be taken, and foods which tend to produce flatulence should be avoided.

Adequate relaxed and restful sleep is essential and this can be helped by a quiet mind. So many problems can be solved by the mere fact of thinking aloud or talking them out with a sympathetic listener.

Two Associations offer very helpful advice in the form of leaflets and pamphlets, and these can be obtained from:

The Heart Foundation Appeal (British), 57 Gloucester Place, London W1., and

The Chest and Heart Association, Tavistock House North, Tavistock Square, London WC1.

Abdominal surgery

The list of surgical operations which can be performed on the stomach, guts, childbearing and sex organs is long and every operation cannot be included in this book.

General treatment of patients after abdominal operations also varies according to the surgeon performing the operation. Therefore it is important that adequate instruction and advice is received before the patient is brought home. It is wise to make a list of questions as you think of them when the patient is in hospital, otherwise it will be difficult to think of them on discharge day!

Patients who have had part of their stomachs removed will have a much smaller capacity for food and drink and therefore should be given frequent small meals and feeds.

Those who have had an operation on their gall-bladder for inflammation may need a low-fat diet, whilst those who have had gall-stones removed will be able to eat normal food.

Some patients who have had a simple removal of appendix will be able to eat a normal diet almost immediately, but if

173

a chronic or 'grumbling' appendix was the trouble, a lighter diet may be ordered for a while.

A patient who has had the prostate gland removed may experience some difficulty in passing or controlling the passing of his water. It is helpful to give him plenty of fluids and to encourage him to pass water at two-hourly intervals for the first week or so.

Advice may be needed on sexual intercourse, especially if a gynaecological operation has been performed. There is no reason, however, why a patient who has had a straightforward hysterectomy should not resume a full sex life.

Care should be taken after abdominal operations when lifting and reaching, stretching or pulling. Heavy suitcases, for example, should not be carried. Housewives need help with shopping, cleaning and laundering at this time. A rupture occurring along the line of the operation incision can be very difficult to repair. It is for this reason that if the hernia is reducible, an abdominal belt is often prescribed instead of surgery.

Piles (Haemorrhoids)

Internal haemorrhoids are due to the rectal veins becoming varicosed. These venous swellings become congested and are liable to bleed during straining when the bowels are being opened. Constipation is the commonest cause of bleeding.

When haemorrhoids are small they can be treated by an injection (of 5 per cent phenol in almond oil). An aseptic inflammatory reaction causes the haemorrhoids to shrink. When they protrude through the anus all the time, causing irritation and discomfort, an operation is usually necessary.

Following surgery for piles, the patient is usually allowed home in less than a week.

Anal dilatation with a special instrument may have to be continued but the patient will be instructed in the procedure, which he can perform for himself. It is important to keep the bowels moving and Senokot or Normacol may be prescribed. Frequent baths should be taken, especially after the bowels have been opened.

Sometimes – but not often – a haemorrhage occurs eight to ten days after the operation. Usually very little blood is lost, but if this occurs the patient should be put to bed and the family doctor called. If there is profuse loss of blood, the patient may have to be re-admitted to hospital.

Cataract operation

The term 'cataract' means opacity in the crystalline lens of the eye.

Most people over the age of sixty have some degree of lens opacity but only a very small minority require surgery.

Some surgeons give the patient the choice of having the operation performed under a local or a general anaesthetic. After the operation, the upper eyelid is sutured to close the eye, and strapped to the cheek. Gauze is impregnated with vaseline, a pad and a metal shield are applied and held in place with strapping.

After twenty-four hours the sutures are removed and after drops have been instilled the dressings and pad are removed. This procedure is repeated daily until the seventh or eighth day when the patient is discharged home wearing light-weight tinted spectacles. No further covering of the eye is required.

Drops will need to be instilled daily (see Chapter 6) and an appointment to attend the out-patient clinic will be given for two weeks in advance.

The patient should not stoop or carry out any strenuous exercises before this appointment is kept.

Usually about six weeks later the drops are discontinued and the patient is given an optical prescription – for spectacles or contact lens.

Spina bifida

Surgery for this condition has become one of the most common surgical operations performed on babies.

Therapy to control hydrocephalus will be performed and the baby discharged home within one month of birth. By that time the back lesions as well as the incisions required for insertions of the plastic valve and tube will have healed.

It is advisable for the mother to spend a few days in hospital before the infant is brought home. During this time she must get used to handling the baby, learn not to be afraid of it and learn how to express his bladder. It takes a little while to get used to the idea that he has a valve in his head, to learn the symptoms of blockage of the tube and how to look out for them. (The baby must be taken back to hospital should it happen.) It is helpful to get to know the social worker too, and to ask for precise instructions of management from the doctor or ward sister.

It is helpful to many parents of spina bifida children to join the Association of Spina Bifida and Hydrocephalus (ASBAH) and the social worker will give the name of the local secretary. They have many books and pamphlets written for parents and *Link*, the Association's journal, is a useful publication to receive regularly.

Even after surgery there will be multiple handicap, but it is important to realize that these children should lead as full and as normal a life as possible. The majority should be able to attend normal play groups even if they are in calipers or wheelchairs. Many will be able to attend primary schools and normal secondary schools. Residential schooling at a school for the physically handicapped should be regarded as a last resort.

It is important to remember that these infants do not feel pain, heat or cold over the affected parts of their legs. Corrective surgery of the legs may be undertaken at the end of the first year of life.

Tonsillectomy

The tonsils are two lymphatic glands, one on each side of the throat. Their function – together with the adenoids, which are at the back of the nose in the space above the roof of the mouth – is to drain the infected material which collects in the nose and throat into the glands at the side of the neck. Sometimes the tonsils (and adenoids) themselves become infected and if the child gets repeated attacks of tonsilitis, the family doctor may advise that the tonsils (often together with the adenoids) should be removed. Great thought should be given to the decision to operate as it is not a simple procedure. Often at the age of seven to nine (when the nose begins to grow and the child does not have to breathe through his mouth every time he gets a cold) there is natural recovery from these recurrent attacks.

After tonsillectomy, the throat is sometimes sore, and soft cold food – especially ice cream – and plenty of drinks should be given. Some doctors prescribe an emulsion which contains a mild pain killer if the soreness is severe. If bleeding occurs, the doctor should be informed at once.

14. Nursing a dying person

The majority of patients suffering from fatal illnesses are nursed in their own homes.

Good nursing care is essential, for whereas recovery from acute illnesses rests upon two essentials, i.e. care by the nurse and cure by the physician, in cases of fatal illness nursing care is the only treatment.

The aims should be (a) freedom from fear, (b) freedom from pain, and (c) cleanliness.

Feeding

Feeding must be adequate and suitable. Normal utensils should be used whenever possible.

Small, frequent, easily digested feeds or nourishing drinks should be given between meals to avoid thirst, hunger or a feeling of tiredness. If possible, the diet should not be restricted. If alcohol is usually taken, this should not be discouraged unless so ordered by the family doctor. It is important to keep up an adequate fluid intake so that all systems function as comfortably as possible and the mouth, lips and tongue are kept moist.

(Details of diets including ideas for varying fluids are given in Chapter 5.)

Grooming is also very important.

Grooming and washing

Concepts of cleanliness vary, but a patient's standards should never be lowered because he is sick. (On the contrary, low standards may well be raised during illness.) The number of washings or baths a patient has is determined by his physical needs and by his personal wishes (except in the case of a psychotic patient where compulsions exist). They should be frequent enough to give him the feeling and appearance of cleanliness, to control body odours, and to protect the skin from maceration and other forms of irritation.

A patient should be kept clean regardless of his size, his position, or his physical and emotional state. (See Chapter 4 for detailed description of bathing in bed.)

A time for observing

When bathing a sick adult, child or baby, learn to assess accurately his general physical condition. Observe his colour, his skin, any localized tenderness or suggestion of soreness, whether he appears apathetic or listless, and so on. Report any abnormality.

Listen, explain, and reassure, as well as observe. In order to comfort, you must gain your patient's confidence.

Sickness

Sickness is sometimes a distressing symptom: if it persists, it should be reported. Drugs to prevent vomiting may be ordered.

Whilst the patient is being sick, support his head with your left hand and, with your right, hold a receiver or bowl for him to be sick into.

As soon as the vomiting attack is over a mouthwash should be given and the patient's face sponged with warm water and dried gently.

Soiled linen or clothing must be changed and cleaned immediately.

Giving medicines

All medicines must be given at the correct time (see Chapter 6). During painful illnesses, pain killers should be given before pain sets in, and the doctor will ask you to see that they are given at regular intervals to ensure this.

The control of pain is a very complex procedure and a patient's personality should not be altered because of it. It is important, therefore, to find the drug which suits him best and which enables him to retain his faculties whilst being mentally composed: so note and report to the doctor the reactions of your patient to any medicine or drug you give him. Indeed, any physical, mental, or emotional change should be observed and reported.

Positioning

The positions used in nursing vary with the needs of the patient. As a rule, patients lying in bed are nursed in the recumbent or semi-recumbent position. The best position is the one the patient finds most comfortable: otherwise it must be one which will enable his limbs and organs to function to their maximum capacity and, if feasible, to be restored with complete function.

The dorsal recumbent or supine position provides for full relaxation and is the one in which many acutely ill patients are nursed. The patient lies on his back with one soft pillow, and his knees very slightly flexed.

The recovery, or post-operative 'tonsil' position is an exaggerated semi-prone position used for an unconscious patient. His trunk is almost prone, his right arm flexed, his left arm lying beside his body. His right leg is flexed in front of him to give him stability (see page 20 for diagram).

An unconscious or paralysed patient must be moved frequently. Healthy people move constantly even in sleep, and a patient who is unable to move himself should not be left in one position for more than two hours. The strictest attention to all pressure areas is essential when helping to care for a helpless patient.

Loneliness in illness

Loneliness in serious illness can be the determining cause of death particularly in old people and young children.

It is extremely important to be constantly with a very ill patient – touch him, hold his hand, speak to him – and listen.

Relieve obvious discomforts he cannot express – give him a drink, plump his pillow, move his head, wipe away the sweat, push the hair away from his eyes. If he is unable to swallow, moisten his lips and mouth; sponge his hands and face: alter his position to prevent sores or cramp; raise his shoulders to relieve his breathing. Do not run away. In other words, observe his needs – and meet them without them being expressed.

Incontinence

Failure to control the bladder or the bowel is unpleasant for the patient and for the nurse.

Incontinence of urine can often be prevented by giving a bedpan or urinal at regular intervals – e.g. every two hours.

A regular bowel action can often be achieved by giving a diet containing fruit and vegetables, and as much fluid as possible.

A suppository may be ordered daily or on alternate days (see page 68 for details of how to administer these).

If incontinence occurs, the bed and clothing must be changed immediately. The skin should be washed with soap and water *and carefully dried.* A barrier cream, giving a waterproof covering, may be used.

Disposable incontinence pads are available from your nurse, or can be bought from most chemists.

In some areas there is a laundry service provided under the National Health Service.

Incontinent old people are often very distressed by their condition and should be treated with compassion and understanding, patience and sympathy.

Sleeplessness (insomnia)

Discomfort and pain are probably the most frequent causes of sleeplessness.

Discomfort can be due to an uncomfortable position, an uncomfortable bed, a wrinkled bottom sheet, or the weight of clothes needing adjustment; or it can be localized personal discomfort, e.g. a too-tight dressing, or plaster, pressure, or a skin irritation. All these have obvious remedies.

Indigestion, a common cause of sleeplessness, can be

alleviated by hot peppermint water or by one of the commercial brands of 'dyspepsia tablets'.

Nausea sometimes responds to soda water, bicarbonate of soda in water, or tonic water; headaches, to the simple non-aspirin analgesics on the market (if allowed by your patient's nurse or doctor).

If discomfort is caused by perspiration, warm sponging and careful drying, followed by a complete change of night clothes and bedclothes, will be necessary.

The sense of smell is especially acute when the body is sick, and it is important to prevent unpleasant smells penetrating the sick room for instance, the smell of cooking. Leave an aerosol within easy reach of your patient. This is especially necessary if he has a discharging wound. Remember that an unpleasant smell which may be hardly noticeable to you can be a source of displeasure and therefore cause restlessness to a patient who is trying to get to sleep.

It would seem obvious to make sure that your patient has either been accompanied to the lavatory or has been offered a bedpan or urinal before settling down for the night, but this is sometimes forgotten and the discomfort prevents sleep.

There are, of course, many other causes of discomfort, but always the accent should be on preventing them: think ahead, and try to forstall every likely situation.

Hunger and thirst

These are easily remedied if your patient is allowed to take whatever he likes, but try to ensure that he has an adequate light diet and fluids before resting. If, in spite of this, he is likely to wake in the night feeling hungry, leave a milk drink in a thermos on the bedside table (in addition to a jug of water or fruit juice). If your patient is not allowed to drink, he may like a boiled sweet to suck. Also see that he has frequent opportunities to clean his mouth and teeth – soda or tonic water make refreshing mouthwashes. It may be necessary to clean his mouth for him and to keep his lips moistened (see page 43 for details).

Cold and heat

If the sick room is too cold and a fire is necessary, do see that it is well guarded. If your patient is cold, warmer night clothes and additional bed clothes should be provided. *Duvets*, or continental quilts, are not as heavy as blankets. The latter tend to impair already impaired circulation. If bed warmers are used, take great care not to burn your patient. Hot-water bottles must be well protected. If electric pads or blankets are used the maker's instructions must be read and carefully obeyed.

Some older people like wearing bedsocks, mittens, bedjackets and shawls. Quilted bedjackets are the warmest covering for shoulders and back. See that these are within easy reach in case they are needed for the cooler hours of the night. Hot milk or soup make a warming and soothing bedtime drink, but tea and coffee should be avoided. If the room is too hot and the windows are left open, protect the patient from draughts by using a draped clothes-horse as an improvised screen. Again, carefully adjust your patient's clothes and his bed clothes so that he is comfortable. A small electric fan can be useful. Air can be made to circulate more freely around the patient if the top bedclothes are arranged over a bedcradle. If he is very hot and sticky, warm sponging and a complete change of clothes will make him more comfortable, and help induce sleep.

Noise and light

Most people sleep better in the dark so, if it is necessary to have a light shade it by placing a cloth or duster over the lampshade. During the day, if the curtains or blinds are inadequate, give him an eye shade made of soft material. These are also useful when a street light is bothersome, or when a stronger light has to be kept on at night.

Family and friends should be instructed to walk, and talk, quietly. Noisy doors or rattling windows must be attended to, as also must regular noises such as a dripping tap. Often it is small things like these which can be so irritating, and prevent sleep. When a louder and uncontrollable noise invades the room, e.g. the sound of traffic, cotton wool ear plugs are fairly effective. At least, they muffle the sound of horns and brakes!

Restlessness

Sometimes, in spite of every effort being made, sleep will still not come to your patient. This is very often due to the body not being tired, or the mind being too active. To relax the body, gentle, slow exercises, massage, or rhythmic hair brushing are sometimes effective, and certainly worth trying. If allowed, and if it is possible, a warm sponging may help.

For the too-active mind, it is worth spending some time with your patient to find out what thoughts are keeping him awake and see if you can help (without 'prying', and only if he wishes to talk about them, of course). He may be worrying about his condition, or treatment, or it may be that a member of his family is causing him anxiety and all that is needed is a telephone call to put his mind at rest.

Sometimes a long talk is necessary if decisions and plans for the future are to be made, but it will be time very well spent, even if you act only as a listening-post and make little verbal contribution to the conversation!

There are, of course, many other reasons for restlessness and sleeplessness. So, as you nurse your patient, try to find out why he is not sleeping – inevitably, it will be something to do with his personal circumstances or his personal condition.

But whatever the cause, elimination of it should be your aim. Lastly, remember the soporific effect of the 'juice of the grape'. If your patient is allowed it, and enjoys it, a glass of red wine is often effective in producing a good night's sleep.

Breathlessness

Sometimes very ill people experience breathlessness – for a variety of reasons. Dyspnoea means difficult, painful or, at least, uncomfortable breathing. It may be due to a wide variety of causes, including pressure or obstruction on the windpipe or tubes of the lung by blood, mucus, foreign body, tumour, glands, swellings, or stricture. It may also be due to paralysis of the respiratory muscles, to diminished lung capacity, or to heart failure due to disease of the heart or acute disease of the lung.

The breathless patient is often frightened, and it is essential that understanding, compassion, reassurance and encouragement are given.

The patient will be able to breathe more easily if propped up in the sitting position. Even in hospital where special beds are available, it requires nursing skill – and time – to find a comfortable position for the very breathless patient. The patient's head and back should be fully supported by a back rest and several pillows (with no hollows between the pillows). A foot-rest will prevent him slipping down the bed.

When dyspnoea is marked, the breathing muscles are continually in action. If a bedtable is provided the patient may lean forward, supporting himself with his elbows resting on the table, and this will ensure easier movement by fixing the shoulder muscles. In some instances of severe dyspnoea where there are nodding movements of the head, a head-rest upon which the patient may lay his forehead will add greatly to his comfort. A rubber, foam, water or air-ring pillow will protect the bottom of his back from pressure.

Some very breathless patients are often better nursed in an armchair. The legs and feet may be put up at intervals during the day to prevent swelling.

It should be remembered that a breathless patient is a restless patient and will need to change his position frequently.

Because a change in temperature will make breathing and coughing more distressing, the temperature of the patient's room should be kept fairly constant. Bedclothes may need to be adjusted and clothes should be loose with no neck or chest restrictions.

Oxygen should be given only under the supervision of a qualified nurse. Remember it is highly inflammable and no light, cigarette or fire should be used anywhere near.

A dry, irritating, ineffective and unproductive cough may be suppressed by sipping water or fruit juice, or by sucking a sweet or pastille. On the other hand, a productive cough (one which results in expectoration) should be encouraged. Sputum should never be swallowed, and when nursing a very ill patient it may be necessary to remove the sputum from his mouth. Paper handkerchiefs or tissues should be used, and a disposable container be within the patient's reach. Because coughing and expectorating can be distressing and exhausting to the patient, you may need to hold the container for him, and allow him to rest his head on your outstretched hand during an attack. It may also be necessary to wipe away sticky sputum from his lips.

Sometimes, coughing is painful to the patient, and then you must encourage him to expectorate and not suppress the attack. You can further help by supporting his chest for him or, if surgery has been performed, by placing your hand firmly but gently over the wound.

To clear the air passages of patients who have inflammation of the windpipe, steam inhalations are sometimes used. Stand beside the patient, steadying the inhaler for him. A long mouthpiece should be given to the dyspnoeic patient when a Nelson's inhaler is used (see page 69). Although the longer mouthpiece has disadvantages, such as the water vapour cooling a little before it reaches the patient, and the long, unprotected stem becoming hot to touch, it has the distinct advantage of avoiding painful and distressing stooping by the patient. It should be placed either on a table beside the patient who is sitting in a chair or on a bedtable if he is in bed. *Never* leave an ill person alone when he is having an inhalation.

When there is need to humidify the atmosphere of a room, the Croupaire (a special device for babies with croup) or a therapeutic pressurized aerosol may be used, but only if ordered by the nurse or doctor.

A note should be made of food which causes the patient to cough, so that it may be avoided next time. Usually it is the dry, hard foods which aggravate, not the light, moist, easily digested ones. If you have to feed a breathless patient give him only very small mouthfuls at a time, as swallowing is often difficult.

The patient's mouth can become very dry, especially if he breathes through it. A covered drink should be left within easy reach beside him, so that he may take frequent small sips. A mug or a beaker with a handle is easier to manipulate than a glass. If milk drinks are taken, provide water for rinsing the mouth, otherwise sordes will develop. A lip salve should be applied to dry lips. The patient's nasal passages should be kept clear and a bland cream may be smeared around his nostrils to prevent crusting.

It need hardly be added that, in order to prevent a breathless patient becoming even more breathless, all activity should be avoided as far as possible – and this includes talking. Visitors should be limited in time and in number.

How to recognize approaching death

Some patients become unconscious several hours or even days before death.

Others remain conscious, but sight and speech deteriorate. The skin feels cold to the touch, especially the extremities – nose, tips of ears, hands and feet. There may be blueness around the mouth. There may be some perspiring (this should be sponged away with warm water). The pulse volume becomes weaker. The breathing becomes shallow. It may also become noisy. If so, it can be distressing and every effort should be made to relieve it by raising the head and shoulders with an extra pillow, turning the head to one side, or turning the patient over on to his side with pillows behind his back to keep him in position.

Death occurs when breathing and the heart stop.

The patient should not be left alone. As he may not be able to see, he should be spoken to, and touched so that he knows someone is with him.

However close to death you believe your patient to be, continue to carry out all general nursing procedures meticulously, slowly and gently, and continue to talk to him remembering that hearing is the last sense to be lost. Even if he cannot answer or appears to be unconscious, continue to speak to, reassure and comfort your patient.

Protect your patient in his complete and final dependence on you from loss of dignity.

The most precious possessions we have are the spirit, the will to live, a sense of dignity and of individuality. Everyone who tends a sick person should respect the wishes of that person and afford him due consideration. During periods of unconsciousness, prostration, or irreversible illness, this is even more essential. You must also be alert to the things and people which give him physical and spiritual comfort.

Care of the dying is both physical and pastoral: your patient may wish to receive a visit from his minister of religion. Sometimes relatives tend to overlook this need, possibly because they fear that the patient may begin to think his illness is serious but, more often than not, a patient knows quite as much, if not more, about his condition than his family, even if he does not talk about it.

The tendency to belittle or deny death should be discouraged. False cheerfulness is unhelpful. The patient's thoughts and wishes should be conveyed to his family, friends or person most concerned.

If someone who is dying expresses a wish to see a minister of religion he should be sent for, no matter what time of day or night. Do not wait until death is imminent, for then the patient cannot co-operate.

When asking the minister to call it is helpful to tell him if the patient is unconscious or not, whether he can swallow or is being sick, so that he may judge whether to bring Holy Communion. If an unconscious patient regains consciousness, the minister may wish to pay another visit before a further lapse occurs. When a patient dies, the minister should be notified.

15. What to do when someone dies

Laying out the body

Gently remove all pillows, laying the person absolutely flat. Straighten the body, with arms by the side.

Close the eyelids and, if necessary, support the jaw by tying a bandage under it, and securing on top of the head.

Cover the body, including the head, with a sheet.

Inform the family doctor. If he has been in constant attendance and death was expected, there may be no need to telephone him in the middle of the night unless he has asked you to do so. A call first thing in the morning will do instead.

Some doctors make it a practice to see every patient who has died, but if death was expected and came peacefully, the doctor may not feel it necessary.

However, if the body is to be cremated you must tell the doctor. He must then examine the body himself and also arrange for a second doctor to do so.

The nurse will have given you her telephone number and she will come to carry out last offices.

If you are also to help, this is the procedure:

1. The body is gently washed all over, and the nails cleaned.

2. A receiver or bowl is placed between the thighs and the bladder emptied by exerting gentle, steady pressure over the lower part of the abdomen.

3. The vagina and rectum are gently packed to prevent any discharge. A pad of cotton wool is placed under the buttocks in case of leakage of fluid.

4. Any wound from an operation is covered with a dressing and strapping.

5. A clean nightgown (or pair of pyjamas) is put on.

6. The hair is brushed and dressed.

7. Any jewellery, rings, etc., which are to be left on the dead person are gently replaced.

8. The body is covered with a clean sheet and left until the undertakers arrive.

Alternatively, the funeral director may come to collect the body and perform last offices at his establishment if this is requested.

After the body has been removed:

1. Place the mattress and pillows out in the fresh air, if possible.

2. Send bed clothes to the laundry.

3. Leave windows and doors open, so that the room is thoroughly aired.

Statutory responsibilities

The family doctor will certify death and issue a death certificate.

This should be taken to the Registrar's office and the death registered.

If there are any unusual circumstances the death will be reported to the coroner or appropriate authority. (A coroner is a qualified doctor or lawyer, sometimes both. He is appointed by the county or county borough council, but is responsible to the Crown only.) He will then decide if a death certificate can be issued, or whether it is desirable to arrange for a post-mortem examination.

If the coroner wishes to hold an inquest, the certificate of death cannot be issued by the doctor until this has taken place.

Medical certificate of death

The law of this country requires that every death shall be registered. For this, medical evidence of the cause of death must be given either by the family doctor, or by the doctor who looked after the patient during the final illness, and by a coroner.

The doctor is legally bound to issue a medical certificate stating the cause of death even when he is not certain of the precise cause. He then states 'to the best of his knowledge and belief' the cause of death. He also gives the last date on which he saw the patient alive and whether or not another doctor has seen the body. There is no charge for this certificate.

When a death has been reported to the coroner, the Registrar must wait until the coroner advises him before he is authorized to register the death.

Reporting a death to the coroner does not inevitably mean an inquest or a post-mortem examination, although the majority of deaths reported to a coroner do lead to the latter and about one-fifth to an inquest. It is up to each individual coroner to decide what action should be taken.

Post-mortem examination

If the coroner orders a post-mortem examination, no one can appeal against his decision. The coroner's office becomes responsible for the body and it is removed to the mortuary. After the post-mortem examination, unless there is to be an inquest, the body again becomes the responsibility of the family.

The coroner has no duty to inform the family of the results of a post-mortem examination, although in most districts the coroner's office or a policeman will do so. In other areas, the next of kin or undertaker will have to enquire at the registrar's office.

An inquest

Whereas a post-mortem examination is carried out to establish with certainty the medical cause of death, an inquest is held to establish who the deceased was and how, when and where he died.

An inquest is held whenever there are reasonable grounds for suspecting that death was due to unnatural causes, or followed an accident.

No expense need be incurred by the family unless they employ a solicitor. This is advisable if death is a result of an accident or of an occupational disease, as there may be compensation claims to be made.

When the inquest is over, the coroner sends a certificate to the registrar and the death can then be registered.

Registering a death

In this country a death should be registered within five days. Registration can be delayed for a further nine days, but only if the registrar receives, in writing, full particulars, including medical evidence of the cause of death.

The next of kin has to endorse with his signature the information he gives the registrar.

Under English law a death must be registered in the district in which it occurs. A list of names, addresses and telephone numbers of local registrars is often displayed in post offices, public libraries, doctor's surgeries, etc., together with the hours the office is open and the sub-district covered by each.

The procedure takes the form of a question-and-answer interview between the registrar and the informant.

First, the registrar will establish that the death took place in his sub-district (he may not register a death which occurred in an area outside his jurisdiction). He will ask the relationship of the informant to the deceased.

A draft form will then be filled in with details of the informant himself, the date on which the death took place, the address at which it took place and the name and sex of the dead person. *All* names by which the deceased has ever been known should be given so that there is no doubt to whom the particulars refer. The names given should be the same as those on birth and marriage certificates and other relevant documents. This will avoid difficulties in connection with insurance policies, probate, bank accounts and so on.

If a person dies away from his own home, his home address should also be entered. The precise occupation of the deceased should be stated – not just given as 'business work'.

The profession or occupation of a wife or widow at the time of her death should be recorded and, in addition to this, she should also be described as 'the wife of' or 'the widow of'.

An unmarried woman over the age of sixteen should have her occupation described, followed by her marital status (e.g. 'spinster').

The informant should check the draft of the proposed entry carefully as, after it has been signed, alterations can only be made with the authority of the Registrar General. After the signing (which has to be done with special ink, so you must use the registrar's pen and not your own) the registrar will hand you copies of the entry. These will be needed for probate, etc.

Note the number of the entry, the register of the date and the registration district – more copies may be needed later. The registrar will also ask for the dead person's medical card, pension or allowance order book. (Make a note of the number before handing it over as you may need the information later.)

The funeral

In this country bodies are either buried or cremated.

Funeral arrangements can be made through a director of funerals who will, if requested, collect a body from a house and transfer it to his establishment where the last offices may be carried out.

The dead person will then be laid in a chapel or viewing room where relatives and friends may visit and bring flowers.

Ministers, doctors and undertakers are usually most helpful with funeral arrangements. For additional information the book *What to do when someone dies* (published by the Consumer Association, 14 Buckingham Street, London WC2, is recommended).

(*Note:* Some religions have different procedures for the care of their dead and these should be checked upon before touching the dead person.)

16. Helping a mentally ill, disturbed or retarded person

There is a branch of medicine which is called psychiatry and is concerned with three kinds of mental illness:

1. the neuroses or psycho-neuroses
2. the psychoses
3. disorders of intelligence, behaviour and personality

The neuroses

Common illnesses in this group are states of anxiety, obsession, hysteria and some reactive depressions.

A neurotic illness is characterized by the patient's insight into his own condition. He recognizes the need for treatment in himself. His symptoms may appear to be physical, but once investigations have eliminated physical illness, psychological stress caused by difficulties of adjustment, increased responsibility, relationship problems, or family disharmony will be seen.

Anxiety states

The symptoms of anxiety states are fear, inability to concentrate and sleeplessness. There may be feelings of panic or the existence of phobias such as a fear of meeting people, or of making decisions. In turn, the body reacts and physical symptoms such as excessive sweating, diarrhoea, loss of appetite, headaches, shaking of the hands or facial tics may show. The patient often feels very depressed. Psychological treatment will include psychotherapy which consists of counselling, reassurance and making the patient aware of his symptoms. A short period away from the situation which provokes the condition may be necessary and, indeed, prove to be all that is required. A well-balanced diet, exercise, relaxation and sleep will help to restore good physical health.

194

Sedatives, 'tranquillizers' and anti-depressant drugs may be prescribed. These should be administered with care and the patient watched whilst he is taking them to make certain that they are swallowed at the time they are given.

The family's help in removing or at least reducing the problem, whatever it is, is of great importance. The patient must be encouraged to see his friends, make new ones, find new interests, and live a full life.

Obsessional states

In a simple form, an obsessional state may be no more than repeatedly checking that the oven is switched off, or the door locked, but in a severe form it may prevent the housewife from leaving the house in case the cooker is still on or the door left open. In other people it takes the form of ritualistic washing of hands or fear of touching or being touched. These, in their turn, produce feelings of fear, distress and depression.

An obsessional personality is unlikely to be changed. Treatment is therefore aimed at relieving the anxiety. Drugs of the tranquillizer group help to relieve tension, and must be given to the patient at the prescribed times. He must be seen to swallow them.

The support and encouragement of his family is invaluable to this patient and play a very large part in the control of the obsession.

Depressive states

Sometimes the depression associated with a neurotic illness persists and then anti-depressant drugs will be prescribed by the doctor. Encouragement and support of the patient in his activities towards a return to normal life are vitally important.

Hysteria

This usually occurs in a self-centred personality. Many factors are involved, making diagnosis and treatment very complicated. There may be emotional storms and threats of

195

suicide after comparatively minor frustrations. Sleeplessness, amnesia and trance-like states are common in these patients.

It is important that not too much sympathy is given to them. Certainly, sympathetic understanding is required, but it must be coupled with firmness. Stress is usually relieved by psychotherapy and drugs. An adjustment to life and the surroundings must be made – with support and encouragement from family and friends.

The psychoses

This group of illnesses falls into four main headings:

1. Schizophrenia
2. Paranoid states
3. Manic-depressive states
4. Organic psychoses

Schizophrenia

This is a fairly common form of mental illness which develops in adolescents and young adults. It rarely occurs after the age of forty or so.

Visual symptoms are general apathy, loss of interest and initiative, lack of emotional reaction, withdrawal from social contact and impulsive behaviour. There may be thought 'disorders', imagined voices and noises and delusions of being affected by rays or radio waves.

Treatment is given with tranquillizing drugs and is aimed at relieving symptoms and preventing deterioration. In addition, rehabilitation is vital. Occupational, social and recreational activities should be encouraged, and such encouragement may be needed over a very long time.

The family of a schizophrenic patient should try to get him back to normal social habits. Contact with the family doctor must be kept up. Schizophrenics are notorious for relapsing *because* they have not kept in touch with their doctor and have failed to take prescribed drugs. Supervision of medication is a must, and can make all the difference to the patient's life. Unfortunately, even with great care and supervision, readmission to hospital is often necessary, but this is to be preferred to continued treatment in hospital. The aim of professionals and family should be to keep the patient at home.

Paranoid states

These are sometimes associated with the schizophrenic group of illnesses. The onset is usually after the age of forty and the patient invariably has a 'chip-on-the-shoulder' personality. Delusions are fixed and persecutory, the patient believing that people are out to harm him, annoy him, or bear him a grudge. He accuses them of working against him and generally persecuting him.

Manic-depressive psychoses

These include the alternating states of mania and depression. Their chief characteristics are extreme swings in mood, from elation and excitement to profound despair and misery.

The mildest mania, *hypomania,* consists of sustained elation, over-activity and 'flights of fancy'. To the outsider the patient appears lively, talkative, vivacious and generous but his family will probably know this to be a phase during which he is active, irritating and extravagant!

In *acute mania* these symptoms are more marked. There will be acute anger, and grand ideas of wealth, power and position.

Delirious mania is an extreme state following the above states if they are not brought under control. The aim, therefore, is to control the excessive activity and excitement by heavy sedation followed by tranquillizing drugs over a long period. Admission to hospital is often necessary. Here the atmosphere will be quiet and calm with external stimuli kept to a minimum and adequate food and fluids will be maintained in spite of the heavy sedation.

Depression is a sharp contrast to mania. There is a feeling of unhappiness, misery and guilt; movement and thought are retarded. Sometimes there may be complaints of an imagined bodily dysfunction such as an inability to eat. In the acute stage, nursing care of these patients includes strict, but unobtrusive, observation to prevent injury or

197

suicide. Anti-depressant drugs and psychotherapy will be prescribed by the doctor.

The organic psychoses

These include a number of conditions in which there is a dysfunction of the brain or central nervous system with an associated disturbance of the mind.

Examples are cerebro-vascular disease, alcoholism, and the after-effects of some head injuries.

Senile psychosis is a fairly common disorder in the elderly and may consist of depressive, manic or paranoid states. The disintegration of personality associated with dementia is much more common.

Symptoms include loss of memory for recent events, confusion, irritability and restlessness. These old people should not live alone. If they do, self-neglect may lead to a decline in their general condition. However, the strain on a family if it takes on responsibility for an elderly member with this condition is very considerable.

Physical and mental symptoms must be relieved by drugs and attention to diet. Physical and mental rehabilitation can prevent deterioration. In some areas there are day hospitals or day wards where the patient can meet other people thus benefiting themselves and giving some hours of relief to the family at the same time.

Addiction is an organic psychosis which occurs when alcohol or drugs cause mental disturbance as a result of damage to the brain or the nervous system. Alcoholic addiction is a social as well as a health problem. Families have been broken up and the lives of both family and patient severely disrupted because of it. It can also cause severe mental disturbance. Sometimes alcoholism develops as a result of sociable drinking; at other times it is due to the need for a feeling of well-being, and is used as a means of escape from problems and difficulties.

In its mild form, alcoholism can be treated by psychotherapy and social re-education. Organizations such as

Alcoholics Anonymous, 11, Redcliffe Gardens, London SW10 (Tel. no: 01-352 9669) exist to help both the patient and his family.

Severe alcoholism requires treatment in hospital where gradual or sudden withdrawal may be prescribed and carried out. During this period sedatives or tranquillizing drugs will be used. Sometimes nauseating drugs are administered at the same time as alcohol is taken to induce an aversion to it.

Drug addiction. A steep increase has taken place in the use of some drugs despite the legal control of the manufacture, sale and prescribing of cocaine, heroin and morphine, etc. Amphetamine for stimulus, and cannabis and lysergic acid diethylamide (LSD) for psychedelic effects have been used increasingly, particularly by people in the fifteen to twenty-five age range. The taking of these drugs may lead to the more dangerous habits of heroin and cocaine addiction. It is for this reason that if a family suspects one of its young members is a drug-taker, professional help and guidance should be sought at once from the family doctor. Drug-addiction centres where skilled help is available have been established in many hospitals throughout the UK.

Treatment of drug addiction may take the form of maintenance doses to prevent withdrawal symptoms.

Psychotherapy aimed at getting the patient to give up the drug altogether usually has to be intensive and lengthy. During this period, substitute drugs will be prescribed.

The combined efforts of patient, friends, family, doctors, nurses, police and social workers will be needed in the rehabilitation programme. Encouragement and firmness are the keynotes to successful 'weaning' from the drug (see also page 121.)

Puerperal psychosis is a condition which sometimes occurs after childbirth. The mother will be excited and confused and may suffer from delusions, usually caused by a high temperature, toxaemia and exhaustion. The cause must be isolated and treated accordingly.

Sometimes the new mother becomes very depressed or may have a schizophrenic reaction after the birth of her child. It is during this state that the child is often rejected and the mother is liable to commit infanticide (kill her baby). Anti-depressant drugs, and sometimes psychotherapy, will be ordered.

For obvious reasons, close observation is vital and follow-up appointments with the hospital must be kept. If there is any sign of relapse the mother will be re-admitted to hospital without delay.

Disorders of intelligence, behaviour and personality

Mental handicap, like any other type of handicap, may be inborn or acquired. In the majority of instances it arises from hereditary defect or from damage to the child before birth.

The nature of intelligence is not wholly understood. It is highly unlikely that mentally subnormal parents will have children of normal or above average intelligence. On the other hand, however, two very intelligent parents may not have children of equal intelligence.

Down's Syndrome (which used to be called 'mongolism' because of the slant-eyed appearance of the child) is comparatively common. In the UK it occurs roughly once in every six hundred children born. The cause is uncertain, although it has been suggested that an infection acquired by the mother whilst carrying the child is to blame. Certainly, many children with Down's Syndrome are born to older mothers.

Mental defects may be produced by diseases suffered by the mother at certain stages of pregnancy, brain injury during birth (causing cerebral palsy or spastic disease) lack of oxygen supply during birth and the taking of some drugs by the mother during pregnancy or labour. But some can be prevented.

Haemolytic jaundice of the newborn can produce brain injury if not anticipated by Rhesus-testing of the mother during pregnancy, and the undertaking of an exchange transfusion during which all the blood of the child is replaced at birth. (Not all these children are born alive.)

Cretinism, once a fairly common cause of mental defect, is due to a failure of metabolism associated with the thyroid gland. The recently discovered condition of phenylketonuria, also associated with metabolic faults, is fairly rare. But the commonest cause of mental handicap occurring after the newborn period is virus encephalitis. This may be due to viruses which specifically affect the brain or to the encephalitis which sometimes occurs as a complication of a childhood disease, especially measles (see Chapter 10). Bacterial meningitis has virtually disappeared as a cause of severe brain damage in highly developed countries, but where preventive medical services are poor it still rates high. Severe sub-normality is sometimes found in children with spina bifida. Epilepsy is often associated with mental deterioration, some epileptics being mentally subnormal at birth and others becoming so. The reason for the latter is not known except that recurrent fits may cause damage to the brain. However, many epileptic people are of normal or above normal intelligence.

A rare cause of mental handicap is physical injury to the brain caused by a blow or a fall.

It has been suggested that intelligent behaviour depends to a considerable extent on logical and good use made of stored experience, and that this requires:

1. The capacity to store experience.
2. The acquisition of experience to be stored.
3. The storing of that experience in an ordered and connected manner.
4. The ability to draw on that store quickly and effectively.

These are interdependent and if any one is impaired, the value of the others is reduced.

The subnormal category includes those who have poor mental capacity, an IQ of fifty to sixty-nine and a mental age of eight to ten years. This group may include some cases of epilepsy, psychosis, autism or psychopathic disorder.

The treatment of these patients is general physical care, education and training in social habits.

Mental retardation

Mentally retarded children have not developed normally: they have an imperfectly developed or poorly functioning brain. They may also have epilepsy, be spastic, blind, or deaf.

Epilepsy is very common among severely retarded children and less common among moderately retarded people. It can also occur to a lesser degree among people of average or above-average intelligence.

Loss of consciousness and fits associated with epilepsy are due to an abnormal electrical discharge within the brain. Different discharges produce different kinds of fits. The recording of these discharges is called an electro-encephalogram (EEG).

The fits usually begin during the first year of life. They may stop altogether at any age. They may stop, then recur years later. They may last a lifetime.

If fits begin in adult life, they are likely to be due, not to epilepsy, but to some other disease, such as hardening of the arteries of the brain or a brain tumour.

Some, but not all, patients have an 'aura'. That is, they experience a certain collection of symptoms before a fit occurs. They may be moody, depressed, have twitchings, or a headache. During a major fit (grand mal) the patient loses consciousness quickly and may fall to the floor. The muscles go into spasm and for about half a minute the body is held rigid. Because the breathing muscles are tightened, breathing stops. The patient may bite his tongue, wet himself, or open his bowels. It is important to keep his airway clear, and to prevent him from hurting himself.

During the next stage of the fit, the muscles contract in short jerks, the limbs are thrashed about, breathing restarts, but is very noisy, and the patient perspires profusely.He may be confused or sleepy for some time after a fit, and may complain of headache or muscle pains. At a later stage the patient will be unaware of what he is doing. He may become anti-social and aggressive.

In a minor fit (petit mal) the patient loses consciousness only for a second or two. He stops what he is doing, falters, turns pale, recovers quickly and resumes his task with no ill effect.

Patients who have frequent major fits may suffer a change in personality. Some become moody, difficult and even hostile. Preventive medication in the form of anti-convulsive drugs must be taken regularly and punctually.

The intelligence of patients who have petit mal attacks or very infrequent major fits, is not affected.

Cerebral palsy

The majority of spastic children are mentally retarded to some degree. Symptoms are apparent at birth, or very shortly afterwards. The baby may be blue, unable to breathe and have fits. Many die. Those who survive are usually restless, have difficulty in sucking and show stiffness of the affected limbs.

The degree of mental retardation varies from slight to severe. Often these patients are more intelligent than they seem to be because they have difficulty in speaking and in expressing themselves. Most are remarkably cheerful and affectionate. A few are liable to outbursts of violent temper.

Spastic muscles feel very hard and may remain in spasm for the whole of the patient's life. Even in sleep they are not relaxed. Permanent spasm leads to shortening of tendons and so causes deformities. If the face is affected there will be difficulty in speaking and swallowing and saliva may dribble from the mouth. Sometimes, in order to perform a movement such as raising a hand to the mouth, violent, lengthy and complicated contortions of the rest of the body are necessary.

Blindness

Blindness, or impaired vision, often occurs in the mentally retarded child, particularly those affected with Down's Syndrome.

Deafness

Deafness, or impaired hearing, also occurs sometimes in the mentally retarded, but it is vitally important to ascertain that the slowness in learning is not due to straightforward deafness with no mental impairment.

Whenever possible, a mentally retarded child should be looked after at home. Here he should be given love and personal care – but not to the detriment of other children. He should not be kept at the baby-level of development. He must have the stimulus of other children, be toilet-trained, helped to progress to solid food and should be encouraged and praised when a new level of behaviour is reached.

Many parents cannot accept that they have produced a mentally retarded child and suffer agonies of guilt. This is entirely misplaced. Neither should the guilt be transferred to the midwife or obstetrician who delivered the child.

Understanding, help and encouragement are as necessary to the parents as to the child, and assistance is available in several ways.

Infant Welfare Clinics

These provide facilities for children up to the age of five (school age). The function of such clinics is to offer advice to the mother and watch the progress of the child. Any changes, or lack of development, which the mother may not notice, will be picked up and dealt with at the earliest possible stage.

A child thought to be retarded will be referred to an Educational Psychologist for testing and assessment. If the child is only backward, he will be placed in a school for the 'educationally subnormal' (ESN School). If he responds he will, if possible, be transferred to an ordinary school, and kept at that school – just one or two years behind other children of his age in an ordinary school syllabus. If the child does not respond, he may be sent to a Junior Training Centre, where he will play, paint, sing, model and indulge in social, sporting and domestic activites.

Facilities are available for incontinent, deaf or blind children in Special Care Units. Transport may be arranged daily, and your doctor or Health Visitor will advise on what is available locally.

Mentally retarded young people over the age of sixteen who are able to live at home (or in a hostel) can attend a Senior or Adult Training Centre. Here they receive training in social behaviour, are taught simple industrial tasks, domestic activities, music, games and exercises.

A Sheltered Workshop is a factory or workshop where handicapped people do not have to compete with people of greater intelligence or without physical handicap.

There are several voluntary organizations which aim to provide advice, clubs, holidays and outings. These should be contacted.

Habit training

All children, whether normal or mentally retarded, have to be trained in social behaviour, to dress and be clean, to control bladder and bowel movements. The mentally retarded child is slower than a normal child and will need to be trained with patience and perseverance and over a far longer period. The training of a subnormal child should begin at the same age as that of a normal child and not when he is too young to respond. There must be no punishment for failure, but praise for success. Patience is the keynote.

Clothes for these children should be easy to put on: as few fasteners as possible should be used. In dressing and undressing, identical routines should be followed. Simple movements will be learnt more quickly than complicated ones. Garments should be taken off and put on one at a time. Simple bows should be taught. Use a mirror when teaching a child to dress or undress. Stand behind him, making him watch, then copy. Later he may be encouraged to dress with other children, learning from them also.

The mentally retarded child will have difficulty in telling the right foot from the left. Lacing and unlacing shoes and slippers is difficult as these movements require fine control. Shoes with elastic insets instead of laces are therefore more suitable.

Mentally retarded children usually remove the minimum of clothing, and use little water if left to wash themselves. They need to be taught patiently to remove clothes, use a flannel or sponge, run water into a basin or bath, to rinse off soap, not to set the floor awash, and to dry themselves well.

Washing the hands after they have been to the lavatory and before meals must also be taught slowly and patiently until it becomes automatic. (Care must be taken to see that an epileptic child is never left alone in the bath or swimming pool).

The young retarded child will need to be trained to brush and comb his hair. Again, stand behind him in front of a mirror, and get him to imitate your actions. Older girls will need to be taught how to care for their skin and hair and how to apply make-up.

It is extremely difficult to train a mentally retarded child to clean his teeth. He must be taught how, and when, to brush them. There are several good films on the subject which appeal to these children. They will probably show one at the school he attends, but great patience and supervision will be needed at home. Many parents find that electric toothbrushes provide the answer!

Nails must not be forgotten: these children may injure themselves or others if left with scissors or nail files. They will take a long time to learn to care for their own nails, but with patience and perseverance, it can be achieved.

Mealtimes with a severely retarded child can be chaos! It is for this reason that many mothers take the easy way out and keep the child on the bottle for longer than is normal. Spoon-feeding should be started as soon as possible.

A spoon is the most useful and least harmful implement. The child should be taught how to hold it, how to scoop up food with it, and how to transfer the food to his mouth. When this has been mastered, a fork can be introduced, and then a knife. It may take a year or more, and some children may never get beyond the stage of taking semi-solids from a spoon. Severely retarded ones may need to be fed all their lives.

Cups and glasses may be gripped clumsily, and the contents spilled, but the special plastic feeding cups with cover or lid which are now available from most chemists, prevent this to a large extent. Incidentally, if the child is left-handed, he should not be encouraged to use the right hand.

Children should be taught the correct use of a handkerchief as soon as possible – there is less chance of success the longer this lesson is postponed. Some severely retarded children do not respond, and they may try to eat them and choke. Others may put them down the lavatory and block it, so unobtrusive observance is always necessary.

General rules for training mentally retarded or handicapped children

1. Persevere
2. Set a good example
3. Show, rather than tell
4. Keep to a reasonable routine or timetable
5. Teach one thing at a time
6. Listen to, and answer, questions
7. Praise – even slight success

Special needs of special conditions

Down's Syndrome

The child with Down's Syndrome needs activity and stimulation (unless he also has a heart condition). Play with him. He will respond to other children, music and movement.

His skin will be particularly sensitive to irritation and incontinence may cause a severe rash. Pay attention to the skin and note any reaction to a particular brand of soap or talcum powder so that they can be avoided. Barrier creams are useful if the child is incontinent. Regular visits to the lavatory should be paid, e.g. every two hours, to prevent incontinence.

These children are susceptible to catarrh and upper respiratory tract infections, so an even temperature is advisable – with no draughts. They need to be well clothed, even on warm days. Any colds or coughs should receive prompt attention and the family doctor should be informed. Inflammation of the eyes and eyelids is common and can become a chronic condition. It is usually caused by the eyes being rubbed with dirty fingers. These children are affectionate and love cuddling, but infection from them can easily be transferred to other children.

Phenylketonuria

This common, but very severe form of mental handicap,

is treated by a diet low in phenylalamine as soon as the disease is diagnosed – usually within the first few weeks of life. Phenylalamine is present in many foods including milk, and special preparations have to be given to the child. Now that synthetic amino acids are used instead of hydrolysed casein, more palatable and less bulky dietary preparations have become available and these have to be supplemented with vitamins and minerals.

Children who do not respond to treatment by diet are likely to be severely retarded, disagreeable and unco-operative. They often do the opposite of what is required of them. Again, great patience and perseverance is necessary. Your doctor and health visitor will give individual advice.

Autism

Autism, formerly used to describe a symptom, is now known as a schizophrenic syndrome in childhood. Sometimes there is a low IQ but often the child is highly intelligent in some subjects.

Autism is not usually diagnosed until the age of two or later, but sometimes as the condition becomes more apparent a mother will notice that her baby is 'aloof' and that instead of cooing, chuckling, wriggling with delight and making himself ready to be picked up, he is growing up in a world of his own. This lack of interest tends to make the child's mother talk less and less, and he in turn becomes more 'backward'. Many mothers have remembered later that their autistic babies liked having words whispered right into their ears.

Often autistic children scream at night. It may be helpful for the parents to alternate their nights of being asleep and awake, taking it in turns to comfort the baby. If this pre-caution is not taken the child's parents are likely to become tired and irritable and rifts occur in the marriage.

In the early years when the child has few, if any, means of communication, dealing with difficult behaviour is the first priority. Later, communication develops and the main problem then is to teach the child the skills of living and to make him take an interest in constructive activities. On the whole, children tend to repeat behaviour which in the past has been rewarded, and stop behaving in a manner which was not rewarded. So, it is vital to react at once to encourage or reward. Prevent bad behaviour, if possible, but react immediately it starts. If you threaten to 'tell Daddy when he comes home' the child will have forgotten the reason a few moments later and certainly by the time Daddy comes! He will merely learn that Daddy is often cross when he comes home. It will make him unhappy about his father, and have no effect on his difficult behaviour.

Individual advice and guidance can be obtained from your clinic, doctor or health visitor. Parents of an autistic child may find *Autistic Children* by Lorna Wing, M.D., D.P.M., published by Constable, London, very useful and helpful.

Hydrocephaly

A child with this abnormality is born with a large head. The upper part of the head will gradually increase in size, out of all proportion to the face and the rest of the body. If it is very large the child may have to be kept in bed. In this case he should be propped up so that he is able to see what is going on. Great care must be taken when moving him, the weight of the head being taken separately. If he cannot lift his head off the pillow, particular attention must be paid to the pressure areas, especially the back of the head. Diet and general nursing care are important (see Section One).

Education of the mentally retarded child

In addition to habit training, the child should learn simple etiquette, handwork, numbers, words, letters, singing and dancing. He should receive speech training, learn exercises, help with domestic work and, if possible, acquire some general knowledge.

Good manners may take as long to learn as good habits. But 'please' and 'thank you' must be learned, as well as the need to speak when spoken to, to open a door for others, and to stand up when adults enter or leave a room.

Games should make use of colour, shape, texture, sound and size. There are many educational toys designed with this purpose in mind and advice can be sought from the child's teachers. Normal children quickly learn to tell different colours and shapes, but a mentally retarded child will need considerable help and repeated stimulation. Toys should be selected according to age, the use a child can make of them, and safety. Children who tend to put things into their mouths should not be given toys which break easily or may cause them to choke. This applies to plastic toys, those with movable parts, and small objects. Toys with sharp edges are dangerous, as are uninflated balloons which can be sucked in, causing choking. Plastic bags should not be left lying around.

Water and sand are excellent playthings. Children love plasticine, bricks, pencils and paper. Dolls can be used in a 'habit-training' game, and imaginative play can be extended to domestic activities and to going shopping.

Finger painting can lead to tracing patterns and then to the use of a paint brush. Speaking and singing should be encouraged. The repetition of nursery rhymes and songs will enable the child to learn words. Scrapbooks, stencils, transfers and prints give pleasure, and later, sewing or weaving can be introduced. Any achievement in this field should be praised and, if possible, displayed or exhibited at school or home.

Walks are often enjoyed and the collection of flowers provides great pleasure. Mentally retarded children often enjoy swimming and riding and there are special clubs in many districts. Because epileptic children may have a fit whilst in the water, they are usually not allowed to swim without supervision because of the danger of drowning.

If your child is mentally retarded, you have no reason to feel guilty, or to blame other people. Your aim should be to ensure that your child lives as normal a life as possible and remember, there are teachers, social workers, doctors, nurses, employers and voluntary organizations ready and able to help you. You may have a major problem on your hands but you need not face it alone.

17. Care of a person who has a physical disability or defect

Physical disability may be congenital or acquired. Congenital deformities are present at birth. They may be single or multiple, and there are several contributory factors: heredity, injury or disease before birth, congenital dislocation of the hip, etc. The administration of certain drugs during pregnancy may also result in deformities (as was the case in the thalidomide tragedy a few years ago). Other disabilities are picked up during life as the result of an accident or a disease – e.g. acute poliomyelitis.

Everyone needs physical and mental stimulation. Without physical activity muscle strength decreases. We all know that a few days in bed with a heavy cold or flu leaves us feeling weak. Prolonged inactivity has an even more extensive physical effect. Similarly, without mental stimulation a person can become withdrawn and dependent. This must be prevented.

Independence and self-care must be the aim whenever possible. It may often take more time to help a patient learn to feed or dress himself than if you do it for him. But his outlook will be improved and his morale heightened if he is encouraged to do all that he is able to. The more he can do for himself, the more satisfying his life will be – to himself and to others.

The extent of brain damage and the loss of physical function are the major factors which limit ability. Some patients may be able to perform physically but cannot follow a procedure. However, with repeated instruction a habit can often be developed.

Physical problems may include muscular weakness and lack of feeling in one or more limbs; difficulty with balance; poor control of muscles (as in 'spastic' people); getting tired quickly; defects in eyesight; fluid retention in the tissues, and pain.

People paralysed as a result of damage to different areas of the brain have different disabilities. For instance, a

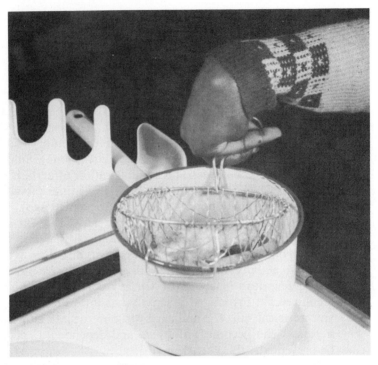

This guard is adjustable to fit most cookers. It prevents saucepans from being tipped over.

patient who is paralysed on the right side after a stroke has damage to the left side of the brain and this usually means difficulty with speech as well. This person will probably have difficulty in remembering and following directions; in finding the words he wants to use in speaking and writing; and in understanding words he reads and hears. He may appear alert and nod 'yes' whilst not understanding you at all. This can be tested by asking some such question as 'Would you like more salt on your ice cream?'

The person who is paralysed on the left side has damage to the right side of his brain. He may be able to talk very well but his behaviour may be confused and he may experience difficulty in understanding complicated spoken or written sentences, in dealing with numbers, dates and arithmetic, and in responding to things on his left side. For example, he may leave all food on the left side of his plate, or shave only the right side of his face.

These symptoms may also occur in elderly people who have a disease of the blood vessels to the brain. The changes in the blood vessels affect several parts of the brain at the same time.

Many people with brain damage, with or without muscular weakness, may have additional signs and symptoms. They may cry and laugh for no reason; they may tire easily, and be unable to perform tasks requiring prolonged effort or concentration; they may show great concern for comparatively minor physical discomforts or may work only when supervised, and be suspicious and irritable.

This can-opener can easily be used with one hand.

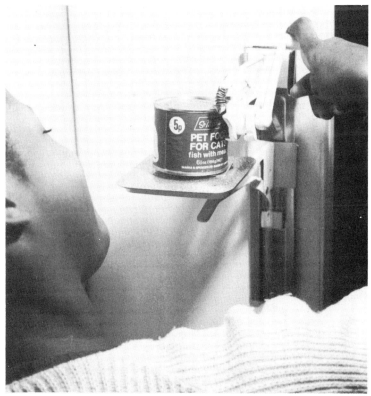

Before beginning to teach self-care you must know what you hope to accomplish. You must also encourage – not as you would encourage a child, nor in a condescending way, but by taking pleasure in his achievements and celebrating success with him.

There are nine points to remember:

1. Know thoroughly the procedure you are trying to teach. Practise it if necessary, e.g. chasing scrambled egg on a plate with a spoon.

2. Know your pupil's abilities and limitations. Do not expect him to achieve something beyond his capacity. Allow him to do what he can. Do not expect him to do things he cannot.

3. Encourage, but do not pressurize, him. Learning new procedures is hard work. Some days he may not be able to do what he has done on previous days. If he has difficulty, help him.

4. Provide proper equipment, enough time, and adequate space so that he practises under conditions as ideal as possible.

5. Adapt procedures to suit your pupil.

6. Ensure that all members of the family know your aims and teach the same procedure in the same way, using the same words and the same stages or steps in a procedure.

7. Teach by using short sentences. Repeat them.

8. Do, rather than tell, whenever possible.

9. Have patience to repeat again and again.

Eating

A paralysed person may need help with cutting up meat, buttering bread and other procedures usually requiring two hands, but after some practice he will be able to achieve these with one hand. If ordinary implements are unsatisfactory a special knife/fork combination may be used. (A list of helpful aids of this kind is obtainable from the British Red Cross Society, Supply Department, 4 Grosvenor Crescent, London SW1X 7EJ.)

If a plate or bowl slides about, a special stand can be used, but a wet dishcloth or wet paper towel usually steadies it.

214

Eating a meal can be a lengthy business for a paralysed person, and special bowls with hot-water containers underneath keep the food hot. These and 'compartment plates', where food can be pushed against the edges making it easier to spoon up, are available (see page 214).

If muscles of the face are affected, chewing may be difficult. Dentures fitted before a stroke may not fit properly afterwards. The family dentist should be consulted. Sometimes food gets stuck between the teeth and cheek of the affected side and, because of the lack of feeling, the patient is unaware of it. This can lead to an infection, so careful cleaning of the teeth and mouth is essential.

Lifting food from the plate to the mouth may be difficult and encouragement needed. A large cloth should be used to protect the chest and lap from dropped food and spilt drinks until this movement is mastered.

Cutting food with one hand

1. *With a fork.* Teach your patient to grasp the handle in his normal hand, turn it so that the eating surface faces him and place his index finger firmly on its upper edge.

He then inserts the side of the fork tip into the meat and rocks the fork slightly from side to side.

After a cut has been made, he lifts the fork and repeats the procedure until a portion of the required size has been severed.

2. *With a knife.* If a knife is preferred, he should grasp the knife handle in his normal hand with the cutting edge facing downwards, placing his index finger firmly on the upper edge of the blade.

He then presses the knife tip into the meat and rocks the knife up and down. After each cut, he lifts the knife and repeats the procedure until a portion has been severed. The knife is then laid down and the fork used to pick up the mouthful.

3. *A knife/fork combination* for both left and right handed use is available and may be preferred because it is always easier to learn a new procedure with a new implement than to learn a new procedure with a familiar implement. The

dull edge may be sharpened if safe use can be ensured. It should be inserted into the mouth only up to the cutting edge.

Buttering bread

Many people can learn to butter bread with one hand. The butter should be soft. Teach your patient to hold the knife so that the flat side is used. He should grasp the handle between thumb and third and fourth fingers. The index finger should rest on top of the blade and the second finger should hold the bread on the plate.

Drinking

All patients should have an adequate fluid intake. In the case of tetraplegic people (paralysed in all four limbs), this is vital, as they will have a self-retaining catheter permanently in the bladder and it is important to prevent their water (urine) from becoming infected and stones being formed in the bladder and kidneys. Even if left alone, sufficient fluid must be left with appropriate drinking straws or tubing in position so that the patient can help himself.

Personal grooming

Washing

A person in a wheelchair will find it easier to wash from a wash basin than to have a bowl brought to him in bed for washing. A nail brush with a suction pad attached to the washbasin will enable him to wash his normal hand and nails.

Where there is spasticity affecting the elbow, hand or shoulder, self-washing will be difficult. As skin irritations are likely to occur under the arm, in the elbow, and within the flexed hand, these areas must be kept scrupulously

A glass set in a frame on a stand makes it easy to have a drink without using one's hands.

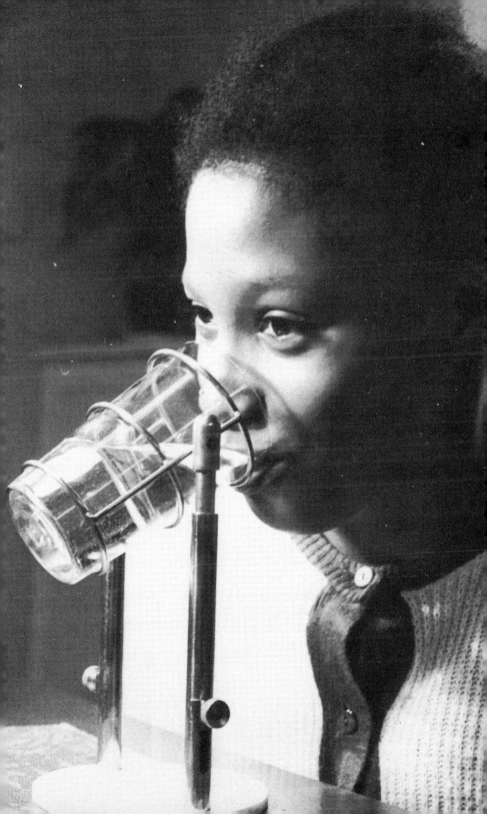

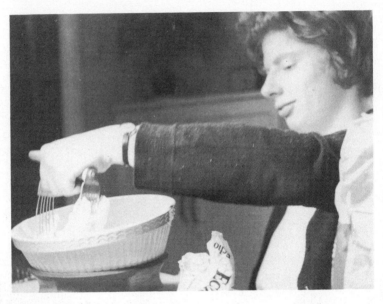

An 'easy to grip' whisk makes mixing and pastry-making a pleasurable task.

clean. If the hand is clenched tight, dead skin may accumulate between the fingers and in the palm. The hand also tends to perspire and must be kept clean and dry. If there is swelling from retained fluid in the tissues, gentle washing is necessary to prevent pain. Physiotherapy will help restore good range of movement and this, in turn, will mean that washing is easier and skin irritation less likely to occur. The armpits and groin require daily washing and an under-arm anti-perspirant should be used.

Careful cleaning, washing and drying after having the bowels opened is important. The care of the skin of people who are incontinent of water or faeces must receive special attention (see page 50).

Bathing

The transfer from wheelchair to bath should be made in a sitting position. Special hoists and rails are available and details of these and other aids, e.g. clothes, can be obtained from the Disabled Living Foundation, 346, Kensington High Street, London W14 8NS.

Because there will be no feeling in the paralysed limb, the temperature of the water must be tested carefully before helping a person into the bath.

One of the main problems in the skin care of people with a physical disability or defect is the prevention of bed sores. Any redness should be watched for as often there is no feeling and a sore can develop very quickly (see page 46).

Care of the mouth

A patient with paralysis of the facial muscles may have difficulty in keeping his mouth and teeth clean. At first

Tapestry can be accomplished by a disabled person with the mouth (a) or the fingers (b) with the help of this embroidery frame which fits securely on to the edge of a table.

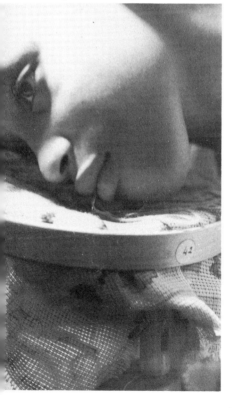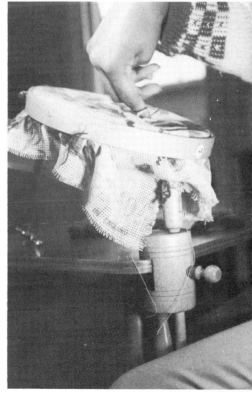

help will be needed, but gradually he may learn to do this for himself. A toothbrush with a small head will be found most helpful but the patient may need some help in holding his lip up and away from the brush on the affected side. An electric toothbrush is very useful for this kind of patient.

Cleaning dentures can be hazardous because of the danger of dropping and breaking them. Filling the handbasin with water will break the fall a little. The patient will find it easier to brush his own dentures if suction pads are attached to a denture brush and it is fixed to the basin.

Early in his recovery your male patient should be encouraged to shave himself with an electric razor. Women should be encouraged to use cosmetics again and here help may be needed, especially if there is spasticity. Whilst many patients are able to brush and comb their hair, it may be necessary to help with styling and certainly with shampooing and setting.

Nails

The tissue of an inactive hand tends to adhere to the tips of the nails. Prevent this by daily cleaning or scrubbing. Fingernails should be kept short, especially if the fingers are flexed, as the nails may dig into the palm of the hand.

Toenails should be cut straight across, and if the patient has sugar diabetes (diabetes mellitus), or his circulation is poor, this should be done by a chiropodist.

Bowel and bladder training

Bowel and bladder problems due to brain damage tend to decrease as the general condition improves. Daily use of glycerine suppositories, and mild laxatives will ensure regularity. Fruit and fruit juice and a bulk-producing diet will help to restore normality. A commode should be used from the beginning – it is far easier than learning to use a bedpan.

Knitting presents no problems to those with only one hand. This aid grasps a knitting needle firmly.

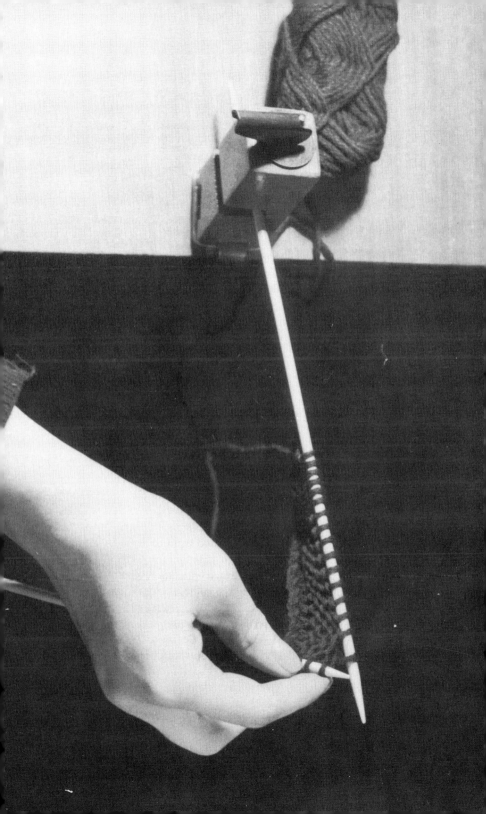

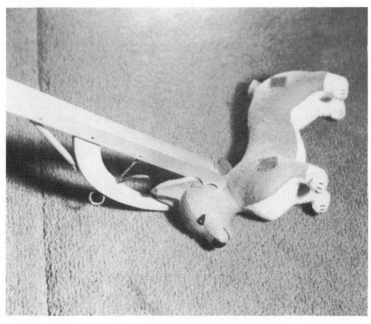

This specially designed 'grab' saves bending down to pick up a toy from the floor.

To begin with, a urinary self-retaining catheter may have to be used and when this is first removed there may be poor control. See that the patient has the opportunity to pass water every two hours or so.

If there is speech difficulty it is particularly important to be aware of this and, indeed, to anticipate it by putting the patient on the commode (or giving him a urinal) at regular two-hourly intervals. If a catheter is left in the bladder, careful cleaning of the area around the catheter is necessary.

If an ordinary lavatory is used, the seat may have to be raised so that the patient is able to raise himself to a standing position again. Details of these special seats can be obtained from the Disabled Living Foundation, or they may be borrowed from the Medical Loan Depot of the local Red Cross or St John Ambulance Brigade.

Handrails are useful in the lavatory and bathroom so that the patient has something to grasp during the transfer from wheelchair to seat.

Dressing

Clothing for disabled and paralysed people should be loose fitting and fasten easily at the front or side – back fastenings should be avoided. If a woman wishes to wear a brassière with a back fastening she should fasten it in front (holding one side in place with the affected arm) and slide it round to the back, put the affected arm through one strap, then her normal arm through the other and gently pull the strap up. To work the strap up the normal arm, she should bend her elbow and raise her arm.

If there is difficulty in pulling up the small tag of a zip fastener a loop should be attached. Large buttons are easier to do up than small ones. To enable a patient to slip his arm through long sleeves with the buttons fastened, sew the buttons on with elastic thread or sew them on to a small piece of elastic.

Velcro fastenings are a boon to disabled people and can be sewn on to any garment. They should be closed during

This card stand allows a disabled player to 'hold' a full hand.

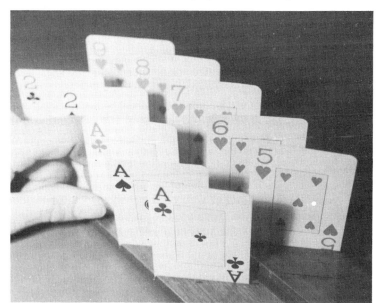

washing to avoid the collection of 'bits' which will prevent the sticking action. Velcro should not be ironed.

Lace-up shoes give firm support for an affected foot and ankle. Socks with loose tops are easier to put on than stretch socks. An angle-top footstool will be found useful when putting on shoes and socks.

Clothes should be placed within easy reach in the order in which they will be put on. When dressing, the patient should begin with the abnormal limb; when undressing, with the normal one.

Special clothing for disabled people is now made. A catalogue *Comfortable Clothes,* published on behalf of the King Edward Hospital Fund for London, may be obtained from Shirley Institute, Didsbury, Manchester M20 8RX.

Positioning and moving

It is vitally important that the patient and his family are taught correct positioning and movements (including transfer from chair to bed, chair to bath, and chair to motor car) by a trained physiotherapist. There are correct ways and procedures, and they should be followed implicitly. If a person who is paralysed on one side is allowed to stay in a curled-up position his joints will tend to become fixed in that position. Such contractures are painful and limit self care and movement. The affected wrist and fingers should be correctly positioned and there are various aids and devices available designed to help achieve this. The functional position of the hand – with the wrist extended – should be maintained. Again, advice from the physiotherapist and help from your health visitor should be followed carefully.

Housekeeping

Many adaptations of wall cookers and working surfaces are available for the paralysed housewife. Help in choosing these is given by the staff of the Disabled Living Foundation.

A specially designed 'straw' enables the disabled to drink without holding the cup to the lips.

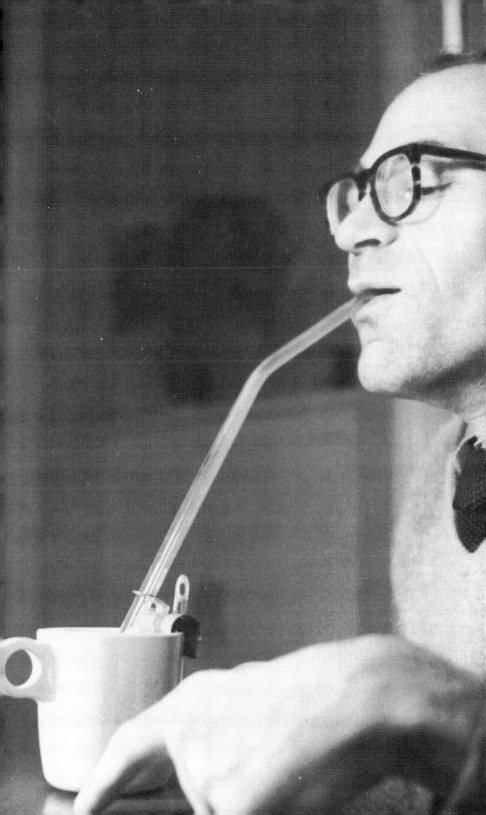

Various devices such as suction bowl-holders, chopping boards, dish mops and egg beaters are available, as also are tap turners, long-handled tongs for retrieving, and so on. The local Red Cross will also advise.

Wheelchairs

Although wheelchairs are, in fact, prescribed by a hospital consultant or a general practitioner, it is often other members of the care team who advise him. Wheelchairs vary in overall width from 22 in to 26 in; in weight from 29 lb to 56 lb; in the rake of the backrest, and in the seat height and depth. They can be self-propelled, attendant-propelled or electrically operated; designed for indoor use, for outdoor use, or for a combination of both. Many accessories such as desk arms, removable foot-rests and arm-rests, and so on are available. It is essential for a suitable chair to be selected – the wrong choice will restrict a person's mobility and reduce his independence. This subject has received a good deal of attention recently and the Society of Industrial

Spiked bread-holder eases slicing problem, reduces risks of accidents.

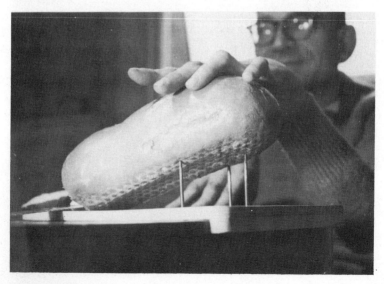

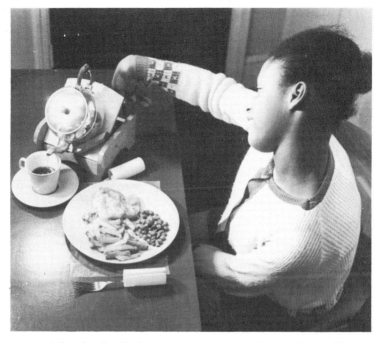

A meal for the disabled can cause many problems unless self-service can be eased.

Artists and Designers Ltd has recently reported the results of their research. Again, the Disabled Living Foundation will be able to advise. The art of using a wheelchair is well described in a pamphlet produced by the British Red Cross entitled *People in Wheelchairs – Hints for Helpers*, and is available from their National Headquarters at 4 Grosvenor Crescent, London SW1X 7EJ.

Hoists

A moderately, or very, disabled person may need some form of lifting equipment. Free-standing hoists must be attendant operated but they have an advantage in that they can be used in many situations whereas fixed overhead hoists, particularly if they are electric, whilst self-operating can only be used under the overhead tracking. The selection of the slings is as important as the selection of the hoist.

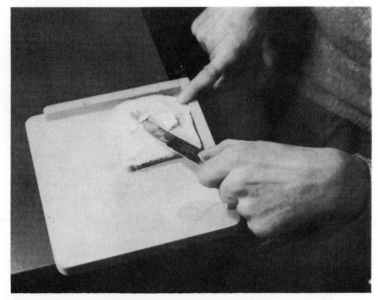

Simple device to facilitate the spreading of a slice of bread.

Many people find that the all-in-one divided leg sling is the safest and the easiest to handle, but alternative designs may be more satisfactory for other people. When acquiring a hoist it is essential to ask for really explicit instructions, and a demonstration of its use.

Reading aids

When difficulty is experienced in handling a book, the correct height and angle of book-rest or cantilever table may be all that is required. A page turner can be obtained (either bought or borrowed, and the Disabled Living Foundation will help here). Alternatively, the patient may wish to subscribe to one of the recorded libraries and enjoy a supply of 'talking books' (see page 233).

Writing aids

Most of us need to be able to write – even if it is only to sign forms. Often the paralysed hand may find the pen too small to grasp and it is a simple matter to provide a larger pen which can be gripped more easily. If the paper slips, some way should be found of holding it steady, by pinning it to a blotter, or stapling it to a piece of cardboard, etc.

An electric typewriter, used in combination with arm supports, or even one of the remote-control typewriters, may be considered necessary, and the doctor should be consulted about this.

Telephone aids

The Post Office can supply a variety of equipment which enables even the very severely disabled to use the telephone independently. The ability to use the telephone is extremely important to someone who is housebound, not only for safety and social reasons but because it may open up possibilities of employment.

Armchairs

There are many armchairs on the market specially designed to give more support for people with a disability. They are higher and have more convenient arms than normal armchairs. Thus it is not difficult to select one that not only suits physical needs but which matches other furniture in the home. Many types of self-rise chairs which assist people (mechanically or electrically) to stand up, are available, and although these are extremely useful for some people, they are issued only in special circumstances. Your doctor should be consulted if you think one would make all the difference to the life of your patient.

Tables

The height of the table top is important as is the amount of knee space necessary to accommodate the foot-rests of a wheelchair, or the stiff legs of an arthritic person. Cantilever tables are useful – they are readily adjustable in height and angle. However, the surface area is small and the design may permit too much 'bounce' to support heavy equipment, such as an electric typewriter, satisfactorily.

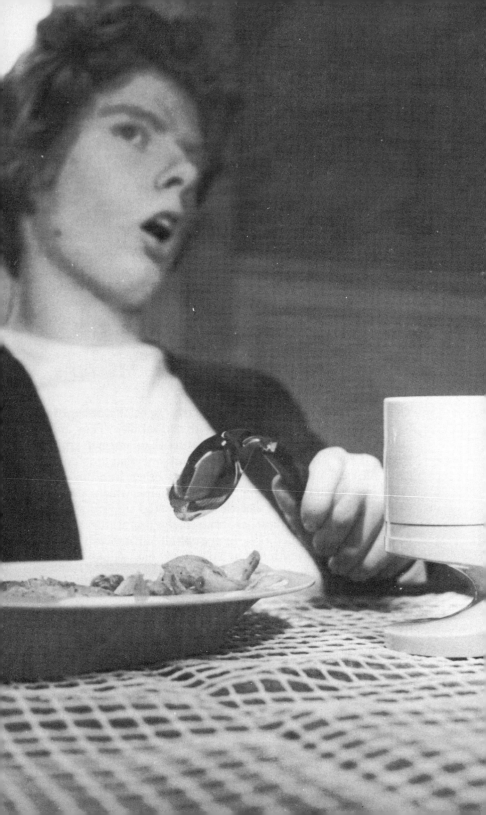

Special gripper spoon helps those who find ordinary cutlery too difficult to use.

Aids for use in the bedroom

There are beds available designed to overcome some of the effects of immobility – beds that sit you up, stand you up, and turn you over. There are also beds that are adjustable in height. In addition to the specially designed beds, there are many rails and supports which can be attached to a normal bed. Bedclothes for a paralysed or arthritic patient are also important. Many people prefer continental quilts, partly because they are so light. People who are unable to turn themselves in bed must have one of the many anti-pressure sore devices. A considerable amount of research has been done in this field, and it is necessary to select the piece of equipment which is most effective for the individual concerned. Advice should be sought from the doctor and from the Disabled Living Foundation.

Thick handled knife/fork helps the disabled to get a grip.

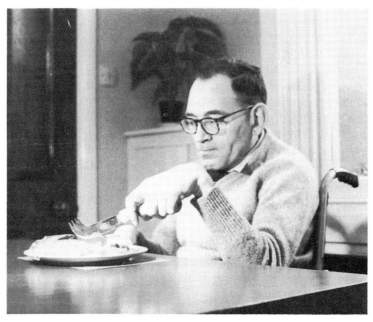

231

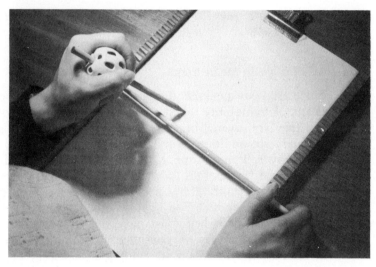

Golf ball pencil grip and home-made guide rule helps the disabled to write and draw.

The deaf person

Patience is needed when dealing with deaf people, and the hard of hearing. Hearing aids should be encouraged, and any early difficulties experienced in using an aid must be overcome. This applies especially to the old and the young. The Possum firm have recently produced a device rather like a battery-operated ear trumpet, and details of this and other electronic controls for the severely disabled can be obtained from Possum Controls Limited, 63 Mandeville Road, Bucks. Quite apart from hearing aids, there are a number of points which should be borne in mind when trying to communicate with a deaf person.

Avoid startling the person when entering a room – normally one hears someone approaching, but deaf people do not have this 'warning'; never approach him from behind; speak in a way which can be clearly understood; come to the point quickly; face the person to whom you are talking; see that your face is in the light not in the shadow; put yourself at the same level (both sit or both stand) so that you each have a clear view of the other's face. If your statement or question is not understood, do not repeat it in exactly the same way – change the words, keeping the same meaning. Do not speak too slowly nor too quickly. Facial expression is 'telling'. Always communicate with a deaf person direct – not through a third member. Nothing is more frustrating or hurtful than being ignored.

RADD, Armstrong Road, Acton, London W3 7JL, have published a leaflet entitled *Silent Night* which gives useful information for deaf – and blind – people and their families.

The blind person

A person who has a visual handicap is unable to identify and approach people he wishes to speak to. You must initiate contact with him. Begin by saying who you are; tell him when you are leaving the room – nothing is worse than being left talking to air! The Royal National Institute for the Blind, Great Portland Street W1, offer an advisory service, and have also run a Talking Books Service for a number of years. This has now led to the formation of a National Library of Talking Books for the Handicapped which provides equipment and Talking Books for all disabled people. The certificate of eligibility for the Service must

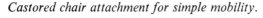

Castored chair attachment for simple mobility.

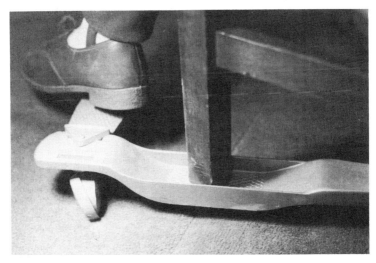

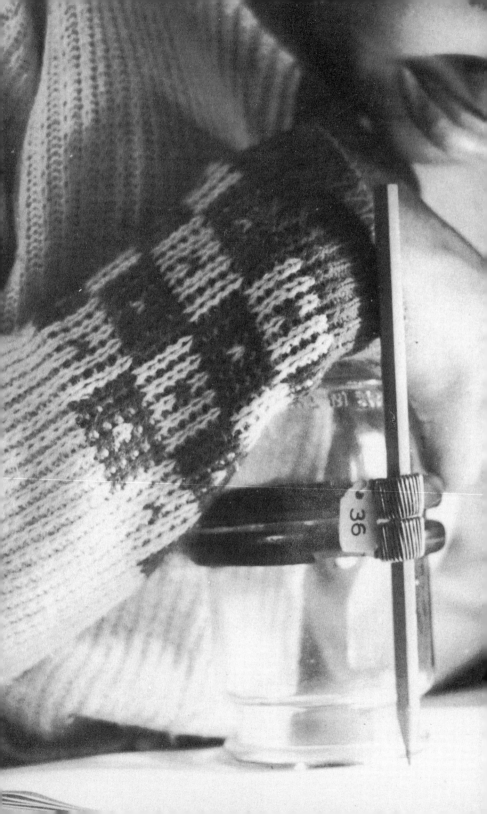

Bands round an upturned jam jar help those who cannot use a pencil normally.

be signed by a doctor, nurse, social worker, or representative of the Society to which the disabled person belongs. Their headquarters are at 49 Great Cumberland Place, London W1. Members must buy a reproducer (which costs about £30–£40) and pay an annual library subscription (£9) which covers the postage as well as the hiring of the cassettes. The tapes are recorded by actors and broadcasters and there is a very wide range of subjects including fiction, fact, biographics, travel, recreational subjects and textbooks for study.

With the passing of the Chronically Sick and Disabled Persons Act, the needs of disabled people have been spotlighted as never before and there are many societies and organizations who provide facilities, services and aids (see Chapter 21).

Convex magnifying screen assists reading for the short-sighted who cannot hold a book.

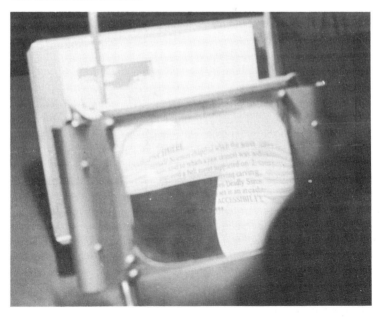

Holidays for the handicapped

The Central Council for the Disabled publishes annually a useful book on hotels and holiday facilities for the physically handicapped person. The book *Holidays for the Physically Disabled* can be obtained from them at 34 Eccleston Square, London SW1V 1PE. *Tel no: 834 0747.*

The British Red Cross Society runs holiday camps for physically disabled people – both adults and children. Enquiries should be made to your local Red Cross or direct to National Headquarters, 9 Grosvenor Crescent, London SW1X 7EJ.

Recommended Reading

Handling the Handicapped, Woodhead-Falkner Ltd. in association with the Chartered Society of Physiotherapy, have produced an excellent guide to the lifting and movement of disabled people.

Section Three
18. Accident prevention in the home

Accidents will happen. There are thousands every year. Many are fatal, even more result in permanent injury, scarring or disability. All bring unnecessary suffering.

Often accidents are caused by carelessness – an unguarded fire, a trailing electric flex, drugs left within reach of a small child, and so on.

Burns and scalds

High on the cause list of serious accidents is fire, and a large number of fires in the home are caused by paraffin heaters. No such heater is one hundred per cent safe but those produced before 1960 are positively dangerous and should be destroyed. The British Standard heaters, enforced in 1960, are safer in design but they must be used with care. Oil stoves should not stand in a draught and should not be moved when alight. Other forms of heating are preferable.

All fires – coal, wood, electric or gas – should be protected by a fire guard if young children or old people are about, or if they are left unattended. If any electric or gas element is exposed this, too, should be 'guarded'. Fire guards should be hooked on to the wall so that they cannot be knocked over or pushed away. The Fire Safety Officer at your local Town Hall will give advice on fires and fire guards and will also be able to indicate other potential fire hazards in your home, such as matches and cigarette lighters left lying about within the reach of small hands.

Clothes made of inflammable material should not be bought for young children or for old people. Billowing garments such as nightgowns are a more dangerous fire risk than pyjamas. By law, ready-made children's nightdresses must be manufactured from flame-resistant material and there is a British Standard test for this.

A mirror should never be hung over a fireplace.

Handles of saucepans, pots and frying pans should not project over the edge of a cooker. A small child can easily grab them or an adult can knock against them and upset the boiling contents over himself. In the same way, teacups and teapot will crash on top of a child if he grabs the hanging edge of a tablecloth.

Falls

Unguarded staircases, open and unguarded windows, loose mats, worn carpets or linoleum, and uneven floor boards, are potential dangers to everyone, especially to the young and old. Non-slip polish should be used on all floors in the home.

To prevent old people from slipping and falling whilst bathing, a rubber mat should be placed in the bath. There are special suction ones available from most large chemists. A bar or rail in the bathroom is an added precaution for elderly people.

Shoes (not slippers) which fit well, and regular visits to the chiropodist will also help the elderly literally to 'keep on their feet'.

Toys and other objects should not be left lying about on the floor or the staircase. Gates can be fitted at the top of the staircase to prevent children and old people falling downstairs. The way from the bedroom to the lavatory or bathroom especially should be kept free of clutter, and a low-watt bulb or night-light can be left burning all night if considered desirable. All halls, staircases and cupboards should be adequately lit. The lavatory used by the very old should also have hand grips fitted.

Remember that old people are more accident-prone because of failing strength, general weakness, unsteadiness, diminished sensory perception, and failing sight and hearing.

With an elderly but ambulant person in the household, ensure that needless accidents do not occur.

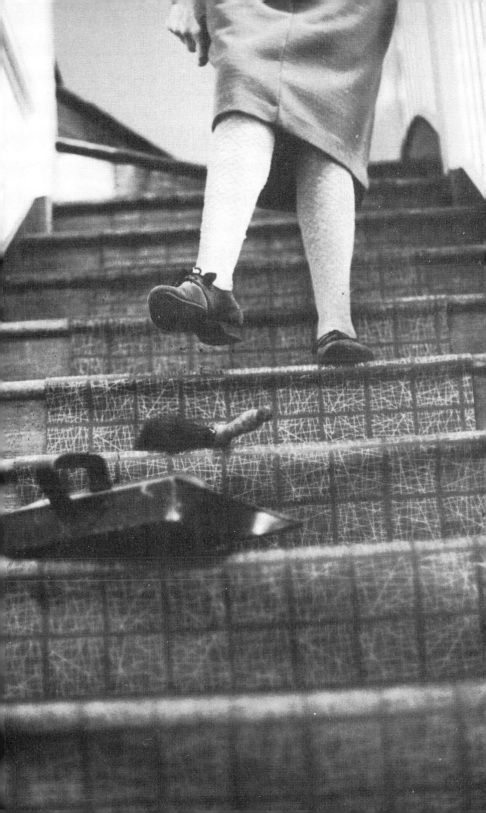

The mentally confused and the paralysed patient

There is an extra duty here to see that the patient does not injure himself. The nurse has to think for the mentally confused, and for the paralysed patient. Care should be taken to see that injury is not caused due to restlessness. If sideboards are necessary it is important to see that your patient does not throw himself against them. Always ascertain, if you can, the cause of restlessness: it may be pain, or an overfull bladder. Physical restraint is to be avoided if possible.

Local applications of heat should not be given. In the case of a paralysed patient it is vital to see, for example, that his foot is not touching a hot radiator. He will not feel the heat and may inflict on himself a severe burn which will take a very long time to heal.

Care should also be taken when giving hot fluids to confused patients. Always stay with *any* patient to whom you have given a steam inhaler.

The effects of exposure

Measures should be taken to protect the eyes and skin from strong sunlight and the extremities from excessive cold.

Excessive cold and heat can cause damage to the skin or body in such a way that tissues locally, or body function generally, may be so seriously affected that death results.

Severe accidental cooling of the body (hypothermia) is especially dangerous in babies and the elderly who lack the ability to regulate their own temperature (see Chapter 7).

Babies must be kept warm and adequately covered during the first few weeks of life, whilst the elderly should be encouraged to eat a well-balanced diet, take warm drinks, and wear shawls, cardigans, mittens, bed socks, etc., as extra coverings during cold weather.

If an elderly person has a fall and is unable to move or summon help his temperature may drop to a dangerous level during the night. Hypothermia sets in if the temperature falls below 32°C. The loss of surface heat is followed by cooling of the deep tissues and organs of the body. This is an extremely dangerous state and often leads to death.

Cot deaths

From time to time babies who appear perfectly all right and are then put down to sleep at night are found dead in the morning. Not long ago, this was thought to have been due to suffocation, the child rolling over face downwards on to the pillow or bedclothes and unable to roll away again. However, modern theories suggest the cause is more likely to be an allergy to an acute virulent respiratory infection. Certainly there is no evidence that parents are in any way to blame. Soft pillows, however, should never be used in prams or cots. Another dangerous habit which causes suffocation is the practice of a mother taking a crying child to her own bed at night. Both may drop off to sleep and the mother roll over on to the baby.

A suffocation hazard of our time is the plastic bag or plastic sheeting. Even those with punched holes should not be left within reach of children.

Heating apparatus in beds and cots
Hot-water bottles

Rubber hot-water bottles should be filled with hot (not boiling) water and placed in a cover. If given to an ill patient the hot-water bottle should be placed between the top blankets. They should never be given to a very ill, mentally confused, paralysed or unconscious patient. Stone bottles should never be used. Care should be taken when filling them (see page 21) to prevent accidents.

Electric pads and blankets

These should be checked regularly and the manufacturers' instructions (on the label attached to each) strictly observed. Care should be taken to ensure that they do not get wet, are never folded, and that pins and needles are not stuck into them. They should be placed in a cover before being put in the bed. The underblanket type must never be switched on whilst the person is lying on it. They should never be given to confused, paralysed or comatosed patients.

Electric appliances

Electric cords trailing across a room can trip people up: frayed flexes on irons, toasters, electric kettles, etc., are very dangerous. Switch off an electric kettle before lifting or carrying it. Switch off an electric toaster before extracting a wedged piece of toast.

All equipment should be tested or checked regularly.

Never do your own electrical repairs – always take the advice of an expert.

Two-pin sockets are a potential danger: properly earthed three-pin ones are safer.

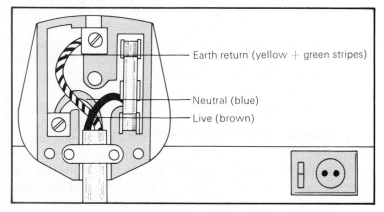

Earth return (yellow + green stripes)

Neutral (blue)
Live (brown)

A properly earthed three-pin plug is safe – two-pin electric sockets are a potential hazard

Sharp objects

Sharp objects such as scissors, knives, razor blades etc., must be kept out of reach of small children. For cutting out paper, small, blunt-edged scissors can be obtained from stationers. Drawing pins, tin tacks, pins and needles should be picked up immediately. Keep a small magnet in the house to make this easier.

Firearms

Firearms must be kept in a locked room. Great care should be taken when cleaning them and this must never be done when young children are present. Children are liable to jump or move quickly, and may cause an adult to jerk his hand. The result can be disastrous.

Poisonings

All medicines, bleaches and disinfectants should be kept well out of the reach of children and mentally ill, confused, deficient or retarded people.

The following household fluids are amongst those which are particularly dangerous:

Ammonia
Antifreeze liquid
Bleaches
Caustic soda
Oven-cleaners
Paint brush restorers
Paint stripper
Pest poisons

Never transfer fluids or medicines from one bottle to another. It is so easy to forget that a 'lemonade' bottle has been used for extra bleaching fluid and other people certainly will not be aware of this. Pills should not be transferred or mixed, even if they are for the same patient and to be taken at the same time.

All medicines should be kept locked in a cupboard if there are children or elderly people in the house. Remember, every medicine is potentially dangerous to these two groups. No tablets are completely safe if large doses are swallowed. When a course of treatment is finished, return the pills to your doctor or nurse or throw them into the lavatory and flush immediately. Do not label them 'for diarrhoea', 'for headache', etc., and store them. The next headache may have a completely different cause. Many drugs lose their potency after a time and are useless after storing.

Poisonous plants, shrubs and trees

If a child swallows berries, seeds or roots of a plant, try to identify the plant. About 200 British plants have certain poisonous constituents but only a few cause a serious illness. Seeds and berries of the following are harmless: hawthorn, lily of the valley, nasturtium, pyracantha, and sweet pea.

The following are dangerous and, if eaten, medical advice should be sought immediately:

Name of plant	Part which is poisonous	Signs/symptoms of poisoning
Aconite	All parts especially seeds and roots	Tightening and burning of mouth and skin. Sickness, loose stools, fits, twitching, collapse.
Berberis	Berries	Purging.
Broom	Only the large are poisonous	Burning in mouth, sickness, loose stools, fits and twitchings.
Cherry	Stones if broken and chewed	General weakness, heaviness of arms and legs, increasing difficulty in breathing, headache, dizziness, sickness, watering of the eyes, irritation of the throat.
Daffodil	Bulb	Sickness and loose stools.
Deadly nightshade	Berries	Confusion, excitability, flushed face, dry mouth, dilated pupils giving a startled appearance, rapid pulse rate.
Elderberry	Leaves and bark	As for broken cherry stones.
Hemlock	Seeds	Rapid breathing, slow pulse rate, dilated pupils, paralysis.

Name of plant	Part which is poisonous	Signs/symptoms of poisoning
Holly	Berries	Sickness, loose stools, sleepiness.
Hydrangea	All parts	As for broken cherry stones.
Laburnum	All parts (Britain's second most poisonous tree). When ripe, poison is concentrated in the seeds, pods and leaves	Burning in mouth, sickness, loose stools, exhaustion, mental confusion, fits leading to coma.
Lupin	Seeds especially. Other parts to a lesser extent	Shallow breathing, twitchings, paralysis, fits leading to collapse.
Marihuana	Leaves	Stimulation of senses, hallucinations, blurred vision, sleepiness, difficulty in walking.
Mistletoe	All parts but the berries especially	Sickness, loose stools, slow pulse rate.
Narcissus	Bulbs	Sickness and loose stools.
Thornapple	Seeds	As for deadly nightshade.
Yew	All parts. Seeds especially poisonous. *This is Britain's most poisonous tree*	Severe stomach pain, sickness, loose stools, paralysis, fits. Death if not dealt with within five minutes.

Street accidents

Many street accidents are not the fault of the motorist.
Children should be taught kerb-drill as soon as they begin

245

to walk. Example is the best way of teaching, and a habit formed in childhood is likely to last a lifetime.

Schools, television and cinemas can also help in teaching road-safety, but the ultimate responsibility must lie with the parents.

See that your child knows he must not run out into the road without looking; dash across the street after a ball or a thrown cap; or run across to the ice-cream vendor or to pick up a conker. Teach him never to hold on to a vehicle – even stationary ones can move off without warning. See that he knows and observes the notices in buses and *never* stands on the platform. Tell him, too, the dangers of boarding or alighting from a moving train. Opening the door of a motor car or of a railway carriage before it has stopped can cause an accident, not only to oneself, but to others.

If he rides a bicycle, adequate instruction must be given on the safety-code. He must also be taught never to hang on to another vehicle whilst freewheeling or to overtake on the wrong side.

19. First aid in the home

(As recommended by The British Red Cross Society, St John Ambulance and St Andrew's Ambulance Association).

Explanatory note

Some of these accidents may not necessarily happen in the home. It is thought important, however, that information should be incorporated in this chapter which would enable a mother to deal with an accident at her front gate, or if she comes across a car accident whilst shopping or taking her children to school.

In the event of an accident or injury it is important that the *total* treatment be given, and it will be found that certain points made succinctly here are covered also in other sections of the book. But the repetition is not made without a purpose. It would not be right to compile a section on first aid in such a way that the reader had to refer – perhaps in a hurry – to other parts of the book.

First aid is the skilled application of accepted principles of treatment in the event of an accident or in the case of sudden illness, using facilities or materials available at the time.

First aid is treatment given in an emergency to:

1. Sustain life.
2. Prevent the condition from becoming worse.
3. Promote recovery.

First aid is the approved method of treatment until medical aid is available.

The essentials of first aid

1. Act quickly, quietly and methodically, giving priority to the most urgent conditions.
2. Ensure there is no further danger to the patient, to others or to yourself.
3. If breathing has stopped, or is failing, clear the airway and, if necessary, start emergency resuscitation.

247

4. Control bleeding.
5. Determine the level of consciousness.
6. Give reassurance.
7. Guard against shock.
8. Position the patient correctly.
9. Before moving the patient, immobilize fractures and large wounds.
10. Arrange without delay for conveyance of the injured person to a hospital.
11. Watch and record any changes in condition.

Do not

Attempt too much.
Allow people to crowd and panic.
Remove clothing unnecessarily.
Give anything by mouth to anyone unconscious, suspected of having an internal injury, or who may need an anaesthetic.

Asthma

Sudden attacks of difficult breathing occur most often at night, and the sufferer has difficulty in forcing air out of his lungs.

Treatment

1. Place the patient in a comfortable position, usually sitting up or leaning forward resting on a table or pillow, but keeping the back straight.
2. Reassure him and provide plenty of fresh air.
3. If the condition does not improve, obtain medical aid or arrange for him to be taken to hospital.

Artificial respiration

There are several methods of artificial respiration. The most effective is mouth-to-mouth (or mouth-to-nose) and this method can be used by almost all age groups and in almost all circumstances except:

When there is severe injury to the face and mouth;
When the casualty is pinned in the face-down position;
If vomiting interferes with respiratory resuscitation.

Vomiting usually occurs when breathing is re-establishing and consciousness is returning.

A person who is asphyxiated to any significant degree will be in a state of unconsciousness. In this state, however brought about, the patient is likely to die – simply because his tongue may have fallen to the back of his throat and blocked his airway. This obstruction may be aggravated by vomit or other matter. The first thing to do therefore with an unconscious person is to check that he is breathing easily. If he is *not*, then the following treatment should be carried out immediately.

Waste no time. Start emergency resuscitation immediately. Every second counts.

Treatment

If the patient is NOT breathing

Support the nape of the neck and press the top of the head so that it is tilted backwards.
Push the chin upwards.

These moves extend the head and neck and lift the tongue forward clear of the airway.

If the patient is capable of breathing this may be all that is necessary; he will gasp and start to breathe. If so, place him in the recovery position (see page 19).

Loosen clothing at neck, chest and waist.
To help his breathing, three or four inflations of the lungs may be useful.

If the patient does not start to breathe after having ensured a good airway. Keep the head tilted backwards and begin mouth-to-mouth (or mouth-to-nose) breathing. This is easier to do when the patient is lying on his back.

249

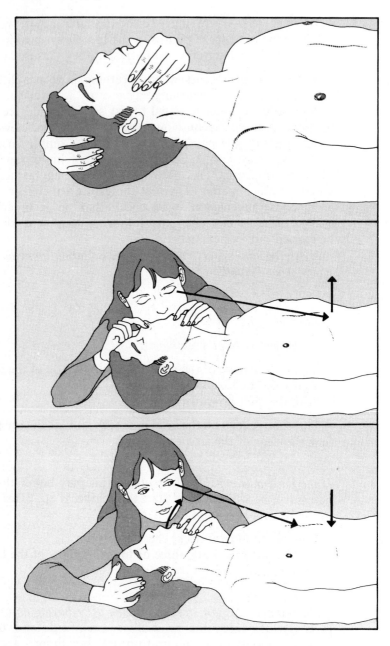

Mouth-to-mouth, or kiss of life, method of artificial respiration

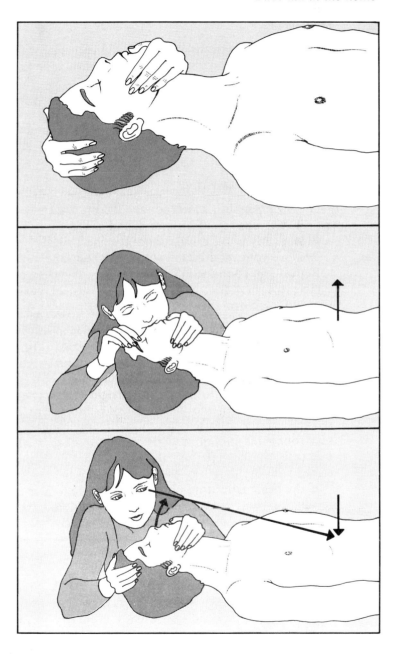

Mouth-to-nose method of artificial respiration

In an adult

Open your mouth wide and take a deep breath.
Pinch the casualty's nostrils together with your fingers.
Seal your lips round his mouth.
Blow into his lungs until the chest rises.
Remove your mouth, and watch the chest fall.
Repeat and continue inflations at your natural rate of breathing.

In an infant or young child

Open your mouth wide and take a deep breath.
Seal your lips round his mouth and nose.
Blow gently into his lungs until the chest rises.
Remove your mouth and watch the chest fall.
Repeat and continue inflations.
Give the first four inflations as rapidly as possible to saturate the blood with oxygen.

If the patient's chest fails to rise, there is an obstruction. Ensure that his head is tilted well backwards, turn him on his side and thump his back. Check for, and remove, any foreign matter from the back of the throat.

It may be easier to obtain an airtight seal between your mouth and that of the patient if his dentures are retained securely in their normal position. If you cannot make a seal round his mouth, use the mouth-to-nose method. In this case, during inflation, the casualty's mouth should be closed with the thumb of the hand holding the lower jaw.

If the heart is beating normally, continue to give artificial respiration until natural breathing is restored. Send for ambulance after placing the patient in the recovery position.

Apoplexy (stroke)

This is due either to bleeding from a ruptured blood vessel into the brain, or the clotting (thrombosis) in a blood vessel of the brain. The condition usually occurs in middle-aged or elderly people suffering from high blood pressure. In a younger person it is due to a weakness in the vessel wall from birth.

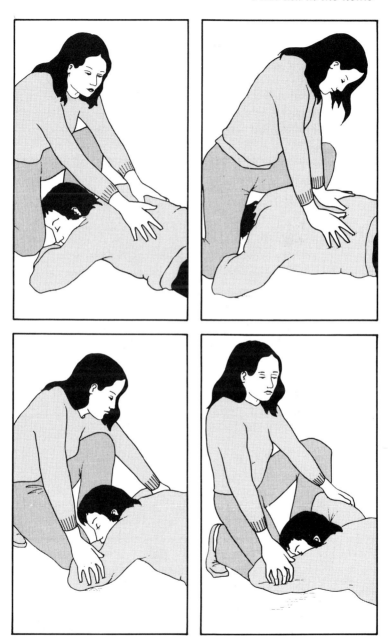

The Holger Nielson method of artificial respiration

Signs and symptoms

These may vary from those of a somewhat less serious nature (sudden loss of power or sensation in a limb, or slurred speech) to serious signs of brain damage.

The sudden onset of the condition, the absence of history or signs of injury, and in some cases the age of the casualty, will help with diagnosis.

Confusion with acute alcoholic poisoning may arise but remember the casualty may have had or been given an alcoholic drink.

Treatment

Carry out the general treatment for unconsciousness, as required.

Bleeding

Bleeding may occur externally or internally and may vary from trivial to severe or fatal.

The body possesses certain built-in mechanisms that tend to stop bleeding spontaneously, and it is important to realise this. For example:

(a) Shed blood will clot, so tending to block the damaged vessel.

(b) The cut ends of a blood vessel will contract, thus diminishing the loss of blood.

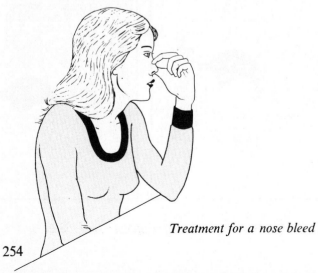

Treatment for a nose bleed

(c) The blood pressure falls and there is consequently less force to push blood out of the vessel.

(d) The skin vessels constrict and reduce bleeding.

Signs and symptoms

As the result of severe loss of blood, external or internal, the following occurs:

Face and lips become pale.
Skin feels cold and clammy.
Casualty feels faint or dizzy.
Pulse is rapid, becoming weaker.
Restlessness increases.
Casualty complains of thirst and of feeling sick.
Breathing becomes shallow, sometimes accompanied by yawning and sighing: casualty may gasp for more air ('air hunger').

These signs and symptoms may vary widely in different persons, in different circumstances, and with the rate of bleeding.

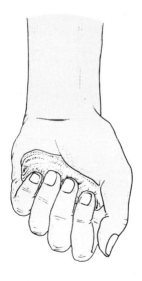

Treatment for bleeding from palm of hand

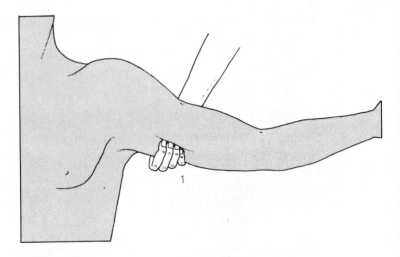

1 Brachial pressure point   2 Femoral pressure point

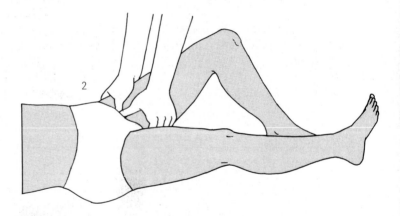

Wounds with slight bleeding (external)

Blood may ooze from all parts of the wound and appear rather alarming, but the bleeding usually stops of its own accord. It is easily controlled by local pressure.

Treatment

1. Reassure patient.
2. Place him at rest.

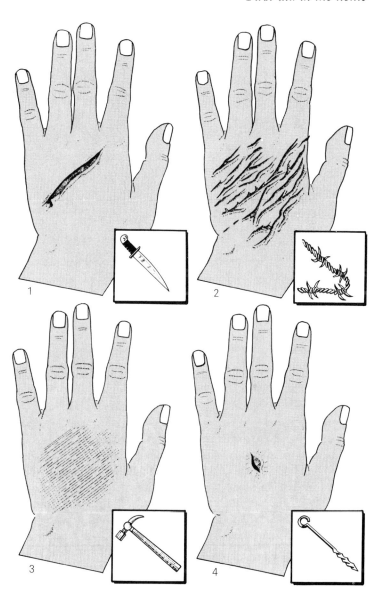

*Types of wounds   1 Incised   2 Lacerated   3 Contused
4 Punctured*

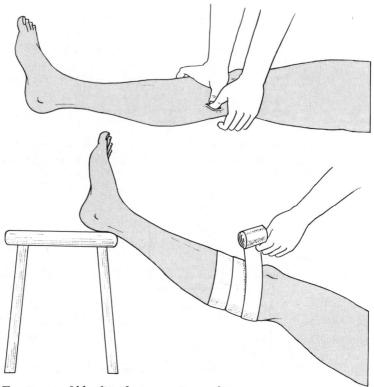

Treatment of bleeding from a varicose ulcer

3. Apply a dressing with a pad if necessary and bandage firmly in position. An adhesive dressing may be suitable.

4. Raise the injured part and support it in position, unless an underlying fracture is suspected.

5. If the wound is dirty, before applying the dressing, if possible, wash the wound with running water from the middle outwards. Temporarily protect the wound with a sterile swab and gently clean the surrounding skin. Dry the skin with swabs of cotton wool, wiping away from the wound and using each swab only once.

Wounds with severe bleeding
Treatment

The aim of first aid here is to stop the bleeding immediately and to obtain medical aid urgently.

1. Apply direct pressure with the fingers to the bleeding point or points, over a dressing if immediately available, for five to fifteen minutes. If the wound area is large, press the sides of the wound firmly but gently together.
2. Lay the casualty down in a suitable and comfortable position, and lower the head if possible.
3. Raise the injured part and support it in position, unless an underlying fracture is suspected.
4. Carefully remove from the wound any foreign bodies which are visible and can easily be picked out or wiped off with a dressing.
5. When a dressing is available:
Apply it directly over the wound and press it firmly down.
Cover it with a pad of soft material.
Retain the dressing and pad in position with a firm bandage.
See that the dressing and pad extend well above the level and beyond the edges of the wound.
If bleeding continues, apply further dressings and pads on top of the original dressing, and bandage more firmly.
6. Immobilize the injured part by a suitable method:
For an upper arm – a sling.
For a lower limb – tying it to its fellow with adequate padding.
7. Remove the casualty carefully to hospital as soon as possible.

Bruise (contusion)

A bruise is bleeding beneath unbroken skin and is often due to a fall or a blow on the surface of the body. It is a minor form of internal bleeding, but can be severe if the area involved is extensive.

The injury is usually accompanied by pain, discolouration and swelling.

Before treatment check there are no further injuries present.

Treatment

1. Put the part at rest in the most comfortable position.
2. Apply a cold application (a cold compress or an ice bag) to reduce swelling and to relieve pain.

259

Cold compress

Soak a thin towel, large handkerchief, piece of flannel, or absorbent cotton wool, in cold water.

Squeeze out the surplus water and apply the compress to the bruised area.

Keep it cool by dripping water on it as required, or replace it by further compresses. Ensure good evaporation by not covering the compress but, if necessary, use open-weave material to keep it in place.

Ice bag

Fill a polythene (or non-porous) bag two-thirds full with crushed ice. Add some common salt to melt the ice and increase the cooling action. Expel the air and tie up the bag. Wrap the bag in a thin towel and apply it carefully to the bruised part. Renew ice and salt as necessary.

Bites

Snake bites

The adder is the only poisonous snake in Britain. Snakes will not usually attack unless stepped on or cornered.

Snake bites are greatly feared, and the fear increases the degree of shock to the casualty. Many persons have died from fright after being bitten.

In those countries where dangerous snakes are common, anti-snake serum is kept available in known centres. If the snake is killed, it should be kept for identification.

Treatment

1. Calm and reassure the casualty and lay him down. Never let him walk about if agitated.
2. Flush the wound with soapy water and wash away all venom that may be around the wound or has oozed from it.
3. Support and immobilize the limb.
4. Obtain medical aid as soon as possible.
5. Should breathing begin to fail commence artificial respiration.

Dog bites
Treat as for a wound using non-touch technique (see Chapter 4). In countries where rabies may be present, all casualties suffering from dog bites should be referred to medical aid for special serum treatment.

Burns and scalds

The effects of burns or scalds are similar and their seriousness depends upon many factors, the most important being the area and extent, rather than the depth, of the injury. However, in young children (especially infants) even small burns should be regarded as serious and hospital treatment sought without delay. The importance of adequate preventive measures cannot be over-emphasized.

The area of most burns and scalds, including the clothing involved, is usually sterile initially and every effort should be made to keep it so.

Types of injury

Superficial – a burn or scald where only the outer layers of the skin are damaged.

Deep – when the whole thickness of the skin, including the nerve endings, is destroyed.

(An extensive superficial burn or scald is more painful than a small deep burn).

BURNS are caused by
Dry heat: fire, flame, contact with hot objects, exposure to sun.

Electricity: an electric current, lightning.

Friction: contact with a revolving wheel (brush burn), a rope or wire.

Corrosive chemicals.

Acids: sulphuric, nitric, hydrochloric.

Alkalis: caustic soda, caustic potash, ammonia solution, quicklime.

Other chemicals: phosphorous, phenol (carbolic acid).

Radiation from X-ray overdose.

SCALDS are caused by
Moist heat: boiling water, a poultice applied too hot, steam, hot oil or tar.

Signs and symptoms

Pain – may be intense, especially with superficial burns.

Redness – followed later by swelling and sometimes blistering; in severe cases, charring.

Shock – there is a great danger from shock which is directly related to the extent of the injury and increases rapidly with the loss of fluid (plasma) oozing from the burned surface, and from the escape of blood or plasma into the tissues causing swelling.

Treatment of burns and scalds

The aim of first aid here is to reduce the local effects of heat; to relieve pain; to prevent infection of the affected area; to replace fluid loss and so lessen shock; and to remove a severely burned or scalded casualty to hospital as quickly as possible.

1. Lessen the spread of heat in the tissues and alleviate pain by placing the part gently under slowly running water or by immersing the part in cool water, keeping it there for at least ten minutes or until the pain ceases. At this early stage reduction of heat is essential, the risk of added infection being of lesser importance.

2. Remove promptly anything of a constrictive nature – rings, bangles, belts and boots, before the parts start to swell.

3. Clothing soaked in boiling water should be carefully removed. Cooled, dry, burned clothing already sterilized by heat need not be removed.

4. Lay the casualty down.

5. Cover the injured part with a dressing – clean sheet, pillow case, etc. With a burn of the face it may be necessary to cut a mask with a hole for breathing.

6. Immobilize a badly burned limb.

7. Give small cold drinks at frequent intervals to a badly burned casualty, if conscious.

8. Arrange for the immediate removal to hospital of all badly burned or scalded casualties as soon as possible, by stretcher if available.

9. Reassurance of the casualty is of great importance at all stages.

DO NOT apply any lotions, ointments or oil dressings.

DO NOT prick blisters, breathe, cough over or touch the burned area, thereby increasing the risk of infection.

Childbirth emergency

General Rules

Send for the midwife or doctor. Meanwhile:
Keep calm.
Let nature take its course.
Do not hurry.

Do not pull on the baby, the cord, or the afterbirth
Let them come naturally.

Do not tie the cord
Until baby and afterbirth are *both* delivered or
the cord has stopped pulsating.

Keep the baby warm

Signs and symptoms of childbirth

Low backache.
A 'show' of blood-stained mucus.
Regular contractions occurring in the lower abdomen.
The 'breaking of the waters' (occasionally).

Outline of treatment

Reassure the expectant mother.
Ensure privacy.
Put her in a quiet place.
Take charge until the midwife or doctor arrives.

Preparation
From the first sign that labour has begun there is plenty of time to get prepared for the baby's arrival.

Don't fuss

Get a cot ready for the baby – a basket, box or drawer. He will need a blanket, shawl or towel to keep him warm. Keep him out of draughts and the cold.

If no sterile ligatures are available boil (ten minutes), or soak in methylated spirit (ten minutes), three pieces of string nine inches long.

These are for tying the cord.

If no bed is available prepare a clean surface for the mother to lie on.

Protect the bed or surface with a sheet of plastic material or newspapers and cover with a clean towel or sheet.

Take a blanket, fold into three, top to bottom, wrap it in a clean sheet, thus making a pack to cover the top half of the mother's body.

Have jugs of hot water available and clean basins, also a plastic or stout paper bag to hold soiled swabs etc.

Prevention of infection

Infection or dirt is a grave danger to mother and baby.

No person who has a cold, sore throat, or septic hands, should help.

Lack of scrupulous cleanliness will jeopardize the life of mother and child.

You and your assistant should wear masks. These can be improvised with a clean handkerchief.

Scrub your nails and wash your hands thoroughly, if possible under running water for four minutes.

Do not dry them.

If they get soiled, wash again.

First stage

The uterus contracts every ten to twenty minutes. Normally this stage may last for several hours.

The contractions are dilating the neck of the uterus and the birth canal.

Signs and symptoms

The 'show' of blood-stained mucus increases.
The cramp-like pains increase and last up to a minute.
As the birth progresses they become more frequent.

Second stage

May start with the 'breaking of the waters' surrounding the baby. A pint or more of water gushes out. This means that the baby is on its way. During the early part of this second stage the mother may be kept on her back. During the contractions she should draw her knees up, holding them with her hands, bend her head forward and hold her breath. She should rest as much as possible between contractions.

Treatment

When a bulge appears –
1. Turn the mother on to her left side.
2. Instruct her to draw her knees up, with her buttocks near to the edge of the bed.
3. Keep her body warm.
4. Support her head with a pillow.

Should a bowel movement occur beware of soiling the birth canal. Wipe clean from in front backwards.

The birth

The mother should not bear down during the contractions; nor hold her breath. She should keep her mouth open and pant i.e. take short breaths, so that the baby may emerge slowly.
The head normally emerges first with the face looking back.
The bottom, foot or arm may appear first.
Do not interfere unless

A membrane is over the face in which case it must be torn.

The cord is around the baby's neck. If this is so, try to ease it over the head or loop it over the shoulder.

Do not pull the baby or the cord. If the cord is pulled and the placenta is torn the baby may bleed to death.

Support the baby's head in the palms of your hands and wait.

The next contraction delivers the baby's shoulders.

Get hold of its body under the armpits and lift the baby towards its mother's abdomen.

Lay the baby by the mother's legs with the head lower than the body.

Ensure that the cord is not stretched.

Immediate care of the baby

Remember that he is wet and very slippery.

1. Wrap a cloth round his ankles.
2. Take a good grip on his legs with one finger between the ankles.
3. Hold him up head downwards.
4. Allow any fluid to drain from his mouth and nose by holding with his head slightly back and opening his mouth.
5. With a clean piece of cloth or gauze gently wipe away any blood or mucus from his mouth and throat.
6. When he cries lay him on his right side close to his mother, not face downwards.

Should he not cry nor show signs of breathing in two minutes, start resuscitation by ventilating his lungs, blowing very gently. On no account should the baby be handled roughly or smacked.

Breech delivery

Should the baby appear bottom first, *no interference* is the rule. Only after the shoulders have emerged and the head retained for three minutes may gentle traction be necessary.

Third stage

The afterbirth will be expelled by uterine contractions and the mother's voluntary efforts.

So turn the mother on her back and separate her legs.

Ten or more minutes may elapse before the afterbirth appears.

If there is much bleeding gently massage the top of the uterus which is found just below the navel – it will stimulate it to contract.

Keep the afterbirth – it is required for checking that it is complete.

Dealing with the cord – leave the cord – do not cut it. The doctor or midwife will deal with this stage.

Care of the mother
Wash the mother and fix a sanitary towel in position.
Give her hot drinks, biscuits, etc.
Encourage her to sleep.
Check her pulse and respiration rates.

Choking

A common incident at all ages. The obstruction to breathing is largely due to spasm.

Signs and symptoms

The casualty may or may not have a fit of coughing. His face and neck are congested and may become livid. Violent and alarming attempts at breathing may be made.

Treatment

The aim of first aid here is to remove any foreign body and relieve the spasm or, if necessary, get air to the lungs past the foreign body if it cannot be removed.

Remove any obvious obstruction – a lump of food, false teeth. If the obstruction is thought to be in the windpipe, in the case of

(a) An infant

Hold the infant up by the legs.

Smack him smartly three or four times between the shoulders. This should dislodge any foreign body.

Give artificial respiration, if necessary.

(b) A child

Lay the child over your knee, head downwards.

Give three or four sharp slaps between the shoulders to dislodge the obstruction.

Give artificial respiration, if necessary.

(c) An adult

Immediately strike him three or four sharp blows between the shoulders.

After clearing any obstruction from the throat, give artificial respiration, if necessary.

Concussion

The brain, like any other tissue, can be damaged. Such damage may result in cerebral concussion.

Concussion is a condition of widespread but temporary disturbance of the working of the brain. 'Brain shaking' is a good description of what occurs. It may be caused by a blow on the head, a fall from a height on to the feet, falling heavily on the lower part of the spine, or a blow on the point of the jaw.

Signs and symptoms

Partial or complete loss of consciousness, lasting usually for a short time.

Shallow breathing.

Shock is also present, so the casualty's face is pale, his skin cold and clammy, and his pulse rapid and weak.

Recovery may be accompanied by nausea and vomiting.

Loss of memory for events immediately before and after the injury is common.

The patient must be seen by a doctor as soon as possible, even when consciousness returns quickly.

Convulsions

Epilepsy

Epilepsy may occur at any age, but usually first appears in young people. People with epilepsy are liable to recurrent attacks, which may be of two types, minor or major; the latter may be due to an addict taking an overdose of a stimulant drug.

Minor epilepsy

The individual turns pale, his eyes become fixed and staring. He is unconscious of his surroundings.

After a short time he may resume his previous activity as though nothing had happened. The condition may resemble a fainting attack and should be treated as such. If the person is known to be subject to such attacks, watch should be kept for the presence of post-epileptic automatism, described under Major epilepsy.

Major epilepsy

This is a true epileptic fit.

The person sometimes has a premonition that he is going to have a fit. He may experience a sense of strangeness, accompanied by a headache, irritability, restlessness or a feeling of lethargy – the 'dreamy state'. These sensations, if they occur, are quite brief.

The fit consists of four stages:

(i) The casualty suddenly loses consciousness and falls to the ground, sometimes with a cry.

(ii) He remains rigid for a few seconds, during which time his face and neck become congested and cyanosed.

(iii) Convulsions, consisting of alternate contraction and relaxation of groups of muscles, begin. There is noisy breathing through clenched jaws. Froth sometimes comes from the mouth and will be blood-stained if the tongue is bitten. He may lose control of the bladder and bowel and pass urine and motions involuntarily (incontinence).

(iv) The casualty then reaches the stage in which his muscles become relaxed (flaccid).

On regaining consciousness, he has loss of memory for recent events and may be dazed and confused and need a little while to pull himself together. He may act in a strange way and wander about without realizing what he is doing (post-epileptic automatism); this condition varies in duration. Subsequently, he may feel exhausted and fall into a deep sleep.

Treatment

The aim of first aid in cases of Major epilepsy is to prevent the casualty, who has no control of himself, from receiving any injury, and to keep his airway clear.

1. Restrain the casualty only as far as is necessary. Forcible restraint of an epileptic may cause injury. Guide, but do not restrict, his movements.

2. Protect him from danger – fire, water, any object against which he might injure himself.

3. As opportunity arises, remove any false teeth and put a knotted handkerchief or similar soft material between his jaws, as far back as possible, to prevent his tongue being bitten. Do not try to prise open his mouth.

4. Wipe away any froth from the mouth.

5. Apply the general treatment of unconsciousness as far as is required.

6. Keep a careful watch for a possible recurrence, and do not leave him until you are satisfied that he is fully aware of his surroundings.

7. Advise him to see his doctor or, if necessary, send him to hospital. Do not arouse the casualty if he has fallen into a deep sleep.

Hysterical fits

These fits usually occur as a reaction to emotional upset or mental stress.

The attack may closely simulate an epileptic fit but is more dramatic and is staged to appeal to a sympathetic audience. The fit varies from a temporary loss of control, during which the person may shout and scream, to a more dramatic effort with arms flying, crying, tearing at the hair or clothes, or rolling on the ground, etc., but taking care not to injure himself.

Treatment

1. Reassure the person gently but firmly.
2. As soon as possible give him something to do.
3. He should be kept under observation and considered as one in need of medical advice when sufficiently recovered.

Convulsions in infants and young children

These sometimes occur as the result of a raised temperature from any cause, such as the onset of an infectious disease or a throat or ear infection.

Signs and symptoms

There may be:
Twitching of muscles of the face and limbs.
Occasional squinting or upturned eyes.
Stiffness or rigidity, with the head and spine arched backwards, and holding of the breath.
Congestion of the face and neck.
Froth may appear at the mouth.

Treatment

1. Ensure a good supply of fresh air.
2. Loosen tight clothing about neck, chest and waist.
3. Place the child in the recovery position. If this is not possible, lay him down with head low and turned to one side.
4. If the child has a high temperature, this may be reduced by tepid sponging.
5. Obtain medical aid.
6. Reassure the child's parents.

Cramp

This is defined as sudden, involuntary and painful contraction of a muscle or group of muscles.

Causes

Poor muscular co-ordination during exercise.
Chilling, as in swimming.
    Excessive loss of salt and body fluids from severe sweating, diarrhoea, or persistent vomiting.

Treatment

The shortened muscles must be stretched.

In the hand. Forcibly, but gently, straighten out the fingers.

In the thigh. Straighten the knee and raise the leg with one hand under the heel while pressing down the knee with the other hand.

In the calf or foot. Straighten the knee and, with the hand, forcibly draw the foot up towards the shin; or straighten the toes and get the casualty to stand on the ball of the foot.

Salt deficiency. Give copious draughts of cold water to which has been added a half teaspoonful of salt to a pint (half a litre) of water.

Diabetes

Diabetes mellitus (sweet or sugar diabetes) is the result of a disturbance of the normal method of using sugar supplies in the body because an internally produced substance from the pancreas (sweetbread) is insufficient. This substance is called insulin.
    Insulin or other drugs are prescribed for a diabetic in a quantity sufficient to keep the blood sugar at normal level.
    The danger for a diabetic under treatment with insulin is that of having more insulin than he needs, because:
    Excessive exercise has already used up the sugar.

Insufficient food has been eaten, e.g. a meal has been delayed or missed.

The person may accidentally have given himself too much insulin.

Insulin coma

This is caused by an excess of insulin.

Signs and symptoms

Pallor.
Profuse sweating.
Rapid pulse.
Shallow breathing (the breath is odourless).
The limbs may tremble.
Confusion – sometimes abnormal aggressiveness, or an appearance of drunkenness.
Faintness or unconsciousness (this develops quickly).

WARNING: The longer a diabetic has been on insulin treatment, the less evident do any warning symptoms become to him.

Diabetic coma

This is due to an inadequate supply of insulin.

Signs and symptoms

Dry skin.
Flushed face.
Deep breathing and sighing. Breath smells strongly of musty apples or nail varnish (acetone).
Casualty passes gradually into a diabetic coma.

There may be uncertainty as to whether the casualty is suffering from excess insulin or lack of it.

Treatment

1. *If conscious* (the casualty can confirm that he is a diabetic).

Don't hesitate. Give drink sweetened with two full table-spoons of sugar or give lumps of sugar, or other sweet substance.

If he improves dramatically, the problem has been one of excess insulin; see that he gets more sugar in case he relapses into a coma. If he does not improve, the giving of sugar will not cause any harm.

2. *If unconscious*

Place in the recovery position.

Arrange for urgent admission to hospital.

Note: The casualty should be searched for a card indicating that he is a diabetic, and for lumps of sugar which are often carried by diabetics on insulin treatment. Marks of recent injections in the arm, thigh, or abdomen may be present.

Electrical injury

The immediate effect of injury resulting from the passage of an electrical current through the body may be extremely severe and cause irregular quivering or tremor of muscles of the heart (fibrillation) or stop its action with cessation of breathing.

High voltage injuries

Contacts with electric currents of up to 400,000 volts from overhead electric cables, conductor rails or electric railways and some industrial currents, may be immediately fatal, or cause some serious injury, including severe burns.

Sudden muscle spasm may throw the casualty with some force away from the point of contact and further injuries, such as broken bones, may result. If this occurs, the casualty should be treated in accordance with the priorities of his injuries. When spasm affects the muscles of the chest, asphyxia may result.

Should the casualty remain in contact with, or in close proximity to, such a high voltage electric current, *no attempt at rescue must be made.*

274

Do not allow anyone within twenty yards. Get someone to contact the police. No safe approach to render first aid can be made until you are absolutely sure that:

The cable or conductor rail is out of service.

It is isolated and earthed near the site of the accident, as it may at any moment, without warning, be re-energized.

Insulating material such as dry wood, clothing etc., is not proof against these high voltages which can jump a considerable gap, thus also causing flash burns.

NEVER climb an electric pylon or pole in anticipation of rendering first aid.

Cranes and other tall objects sometimes foul overhead electric lines. If they remain in contact with or in close proximity to the line, no approach should be made to the casualty until it has been established that it is safe to do so.

When you are officially informed that it is safe, render first aid.

Low voltage injuries

Injury is the result of the passage of an electric current of low voltage from the domestic supply through the body.

Moisture and water conduct electricity and, accordingly, it should be carefully noted that when an attempt is to be made to carry out the rescue of a person in contact with an electric current, care must be taken to avoid direct contact with the casualty, or you yourself will be injured.

Injury may stop the action of the heart and of breathing.

The local effect is a burn which is deeper than its size suggests.

Action

Break the contact: switch the current off, remove the plug, wrench the cable free. If this is impossible, stand on some dry insulating material and, using a piece of dry wood, folded newspaper or rubber, attempt to break the contact by, for example, pushing the casualty's limbs away. Do not touch him with your hands.

Treatment

If necessary, give artificial respiration. Treat burns.

Lightning injury

Lightning may produce similar injuries to those of a high voltage electric current.

Death may occur instantaneously. On being struck by lightning, the casualty is stunned and falls unconscious to the ground. There may be patches of scorching on the skin, burns being deeper where a metallic object, such as a watch, has been carried close to the skin.

Clothing may be set on fire.

Treatment

If necessary, give artificial respiration. Treat burns.

Fainting

Fainting follows a temporary inadequate supply of blood to the brain, frequently caused by some emotional or sensory stimulus. It may begin with a feeling of faintness, or there may be a sudden collapse. Some degree of nerve shock accompanies all injuries.

Causes

A fright, bad news, a horrifying sight, pain.

Fatigue or long periods of sitting or standing in a hot, stuffy atmosphere.

Debilitating illness.

Injury to some part of the body.

Impending faint

There may be some warning before fainting – the person may yawn or sway, feel unsteady, become giddy; his face may become pale or greenish white in colour, and beads of sweat may break out on face, neck and hands.

Treatment of impending faint

1. Reassure the person and urge him to breathe deeply, to flex the muscles of his legs, thighs and buttocks, thus helping the circulation of the blood.
2. Loosen clothing at neck, chest and waist.
3. Lay him down in a current of fresh air until his colour returns, or it may be more convenient to sit him down and lower his head between his knees.
4. On recovery, sips of water may be given.
5. Smelling salts may be useful. Test strength before use.

Signs and symptoms of a faint

The person is unconscious.
His face is pale.
His skin is cold and clammy.
His breathing is shallow.
His pulse is weak and slow at first, but gradually increases in rate.

Treatment of a faint

The aim of first aid here is to get a satisfactory supply of blood to the brain.

1. Lay the person down and deal with any cause. Raise the legs slightly above the level of the head.
2. See that the person concerned has plenty of fresh air and, if necessary, put him into the shade.
3. Loosen clothing at neck, chest and waist.
4. If breathing is difficult, place him in the recovery position.
5. Reassure him as he regains consciousness.
6. Gradually raise him into the sitting position and give sips of water, if requested.

Note: Colour returns to his skin as he starts to recover. If recovery is not rapid and complete, the casualty will require hospital treatment. This is more likely if there is an associated injury.

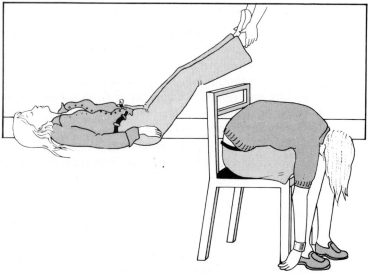

Treatment of impending faints

Foreign body in the eye

All eye injuries are potentially serious, and blows by blunt objects may damage not only the eyelids and the exposed part of the eye but also rupture blood vessels of the eye, the lens and the retina.

Any wounds caused by sharp tools, or even tiny particles which may perforate the eyeball, are potentially serious because of damage which they do mechanically, chemically and by the infection which they may produce.

For all serious injuries to the eye, *immediate medical aid is indicated.* Particles of grit, loose eyelashes, small fragments of metal or glass, etc., may lodge on the eyeball or under the eyelid causing considerable discomfort and inflammation if not speedily removed.

Treatment

    1. Prevent the casualty from rubbing the eye.

    2. Do not attempt to remove the foreign body if it is: On the pupil of the eye.

Embedded or adherent to the eyeball.

Cannot be seen but the eye is inflamed and painful.

In these cases, the following treatment should be given:

(i) Close the eyelids.

(ii) Cover the eye with a soft pad of cotton wool, extending to forehead and cheek and secure lightly in position with a bandage.

(iii) Obtain medical aid.

3. If the foreign body can be seen and is not on the pupil or adherent to the eyeball:

(i) Seat the casualty facing the light, stand in front of him and pull down the lower lid.

(ii) Remove the foreign body with the corner of a clean handkerchief or a wisp of cotton wool which has been soaked in a little water.

4. If the foreign body is under the upper lid, ask the casualty to look down, grasp his eyelashes and pull the upper lid downwards and outwards over the lower lid. The foreign body may thus be dislodged by the lashes of the lower lid. If not, ask the casualty to blink his eye under water.

If still unsuccessful, and if medical aid is not immediately available:

(i) Stand behind the casualty, steadying his head against your chest, and ask him to look down.

(ii) Place a smooth matchstick at the base of the upper lid and press it gently backwards.

(iii) Grasp the lashes and turn the lid over the matchstick, so averting the eyelid.

(iv) Remove the foreign body with the corner of a clean handkerchief or a wisp of cotton wool which has been soaked in a little water.

Injury to the eyeball

Treatment

1. Lay the casualty down at absolute rest.

2. Close the lid and cover the eye with a soft pad of cotton wool, extending to forehead and cheek. Apply a bandage lightly.

3. Remove to hospital as soon as possible.

Foreign body in the stomach

Pins and other small objects, such as coins or buttons, may accidentally be swallowed, especially by young children. Smooth objects need not necessarily cause alarm.

Treatment

    1. Calm the casualty.
    2. Seek medical advice.
Do not give anything by the mouth.

Foreign body in the skin

Treatment

Splinters etc. may be removed with a sterilized needle (one which has been passed through a flame).
    Deeply embedded or complicated objects such as a fish hook should be removed by a nurse or doctor.

Foreign body in the ear

Treatment

Insects: Flood the ear with tepid water or olive oil; the insect will then float out.
    Do not attempt to remove foreign bodies such as beads and beans, but take the casualty (usually a small child) to a doctor or hospital.

Foreign body in the nose

Treatment

1. Instruct the patient to breathe through his mouth.
2. Take the patient to a doctor. Do not attempt to remove the foreign body.

Foreign body in the throat

The aim of first aid here is to remove any foreign body and relieve the spasm or, if necessary, to get air to the lungs past the foreign body if it cannot be removed.

280

Treatment

Remove any obvious obstruction – a lump of food, false teeth etc. If the obstruction is thought to be in the windpipe, in the case of:

(a) An infant

Hold the infant up by the legs.
Smack him smartly three or four times between the shoulders. This should dislodge any foreign body.
Give artificial respiration, if necessary.

(b) A child

Lay the child over your knee, head downwards.
Give three or four sharp slaps between the shoulders to dislodge the obstruction.
Give artificial respiration, if necessary.

How to remove an obstruction in the case of   1 an infant
2 a child

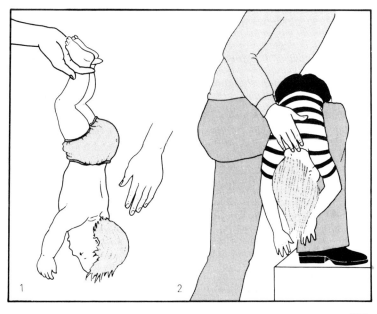

(c) An adult

Immediately strike him three or four sharp blows between the shoulders.

After clearing any obstruction from the throat, give artificial respiration, if necessary.

Fractures

A fracture is a broken or cracked bone.

In young children, the break may be incomplete and is referred to as a greenstick fracture.

All doubtful cases where the diagnosis is uncertain should be regarded as fractures.

Causes of fractures

(a) When the bone breaks at the spot where force is applied. In such cases the force is transmitted along the intervening bones which usually escape injury, e.g. fracture of the collar-bone may result from a fall on the outstretched hand.

(b) When there is a sudden violent contraction of muscles which may cause a fracture, e.g. of the knee-cap or the tip of the elbow.

Types of fractures

Closed – When the skin surface is not broken.

Open – When there is a wound leading down to the fracture, or when the fractured ends protrude through the skin, thus allowing germs to gain access to soft tissues and broken bone.

When there is associated injury to an important structure such as the brain, major blood vessels, nerves, lungs, liver or when associated with a dislocation of a joint, either type of fracture is said to be '*complicated*'.

Signs and symptoms

Pain at or near the site of the fracture, made worse by movement of the injured part.

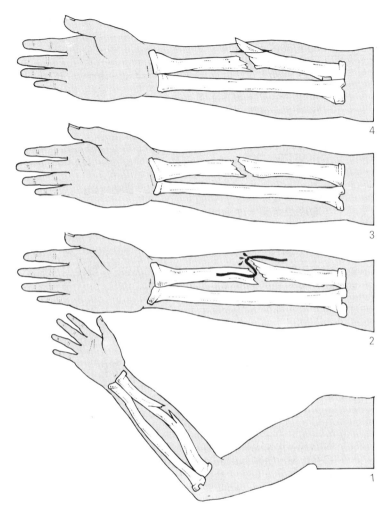

Types of fracture 1 An example of a greenstick fracture
2 An example of a complicated fracture 3 Closed 4 Open

Tenderness on gentle pressure over the affected part.

Swelling, the result of blood loss into the tissues, may later be accompanied by bruising. Swelling may prevent the recognition of other signs, so when in doubt treat as a fracture.

283

Loss of control – the casualty is unable to move the injured part normally.

Deformity – e.g. irregularity of the bone. If the fracture is near the skin, the irregularity may be seen or felt.
– shortening of the limb, due to contraction of the muscles causing the broken ends of the bone to override each other.
– angulation, or rotation, of a limb, due to a fracture of some supporting bone, e.g. if the neck of the femur is fractured the foot falls outwards;
– depression of a flat bone, as in the skull.

Unnatural movement at the seat of the fracture, unless the broken ends are driven into each other.

A coarse bony grating (crepitus) may be felt or heard during the examination of an injured part if the ends of a broken bone move against each other, but this should never deliberately be sought.

Shock – increased by the loss of blood from the circulation.

In addition to the above, the snap of the bone may have been felt or heard. It must also be clearly understood that all the above signs and symptoms may not be present in every fracture. As many signs as possible should be noted by simple observation and without moving any part unnecessarily, as this may cause pain or further damage. Compare the injured and uninjured limbs whenever possible.

General rules for treatment:

1. Asphyxia, bleeding and severe wounds must be dealt with before dealing with any fracture.
2. Treat the fracture on the site of the incident, unless life is endangered (the casualty's or your own), in which case temporary fixation should be carried out before moving the casualty as short a distance as possible.
3. Steady and, if necessary, support the injured part at once to prevent further damage. Maintain this control until the fracture has been immobilized.

4. Immobilize by using:

Body bandages. Using the casualty's body as a means of support will prove adequate for normal purposes.

Splints and bandages. The support of splints may be required when there is a possibility of a long or rough journey before medical aid is available, or in the presence of multiple injuries.

5. Raise the injured part after immobilization if possible, in order to reduce discomfort and swelling.

Use of bandages for fractures:

Bandages should be applied sufficiently firmly to prevent movement but not so tightly as to interfere with the circulation of the blood or to cause pain.

Separate skin surfaces with soft padding before bandaging together, in order to prevent discomfort and chafing of the skin.

Always tie knots over a splint or on the uninjured side. If both lower limbs are injured, tie the knots in front between them.

Check at fifteen-minute intervals to ensure that they are not becoming too tight as a result of swelling of the injured tissues. This is especially important when an elbow has been injured and is supported in a sling.

To pass bandages underneath the casualty if he is lying down, use the natural hollows of the body, e.g. the neck, loins, knees.

Use of splints

If splints are required, they should be:

Sufficiently rigid.

Long enough to immobilize the joint above and below the fracture.

Well padded and wide enough to fit comfortably to the limb.

Applied over clothing.

In emergencies, a splint may be improvised from a walking stick, umbrella, broom handle, a piece of wood, cardboard, or firmly folded newspaper or magazine.

Further treatment

All casualties who have fractures or suspected fractures must be sent to hospital for further attention.

Transport of the casualty should be as gentle as possible.

Special fractures

Jaw and face injuries

Fractures and wounds may be complicated by damage to the brain. The skull or cervical spine may also be injured.

The following serious risks are associated with jaw and face injuries:

1. Obstruction of the casualty's airway with resulting asphyxia by:

The tongue falling to the back of the throat of an unconscious casualty.

Swelling of tissues following the injury.

Displaced and lacerated tissues.

2. Inadequate or absent cough reflex – which allows secretions, blood and foreign material to drain unnoticed into the lungs, causing infection and complications such as collapse of the lungs.

3. Bleeding – which initially may be profuse and alarming, but which is not usually prolonged. It should be controlled by direct pressure.

Fracture of lower jaw

This is always the result of direct force, e.g. a severe blow to the jaw, and there is usually a wound inside the mouth. Usually only one side of the jaw is affected.

Signs and symptoms

Pain: increased by jaw movements or by swallowing.

The casualty has difficulty in speaking.

There is an excessive flow of saliva, which is frequently blood-stained.

Irregularity of the teeth.

Swelling, tenderness and, later, bruising of the face and lower jaw.

Severe bleeding if tongue is injured.

Treatment

The primary aim of first aid in jaw and face injuries is to maintain breathing.

1. Maintain an open airway by ensuring that the tongue has not fallen to the back of the throat and that the mouth is not obstructed.
2. Control bleeding.
3. Remove any false or detached teeth.
4. Support the jaw with a soft pad held in place by hand or by a suitable bandage.
5. The conscious casualty

Not severely injured, may sit up with his head well forward so that any secretions can drain freely.

Severely injured, with downward displacement of the chin and associated soft tissues, may require to be kept in the recovery position.

The unconscious casualty

Must be placed in the recovery position, making sure that the jaw is kept well forward.

6. If the casualty seems likely to vomit, turn his head to the sound side, supporting the jaw with the palm of your hand.
7. Arrange for urgent removal to hospital.

Fracture of spine

This is a grave and serious injury. If the casualty is not correctly handled the spinal cord may be permanently damaged and paralysis result.

Causes of fractures of the spine

Fractures of the spine are caused by:

Direct force e.g.
A fall or a heavy weight across the casualty's back.
A fall from a height on to the back across a bar.
Impact in a collision between vehicles.

Indirect force e.g.

A heavy fall on the feet or buttocks.

A fall on the head from a height (as in diving).

Over-flexing or jerking of the spine as in a collision between vehicles.

The fracture may be complicated by injury to the spinal cord or to the nerves issuing from it, causing complete or partial loss of power (paralysis) and/or sensation in all parts of the body below the site of the injury.

Fracture of the spine should always be suspected in all cases in which there is a history of accident or injury to the vertebral column and the casualty complains of pain in his back.

All such cases must be regarded as serious emergencies and any doubtful case treated as a fracture.

Signs and symptoms

Casualty is found collapsed and complains of severe pain in his back. He sometimes states that he feels cut in half, that his lower limbs are numb, or that he has lost control of them.

Possible loss of power in the limbs. Ask the casualty to:

Move his wrists and ankles.
Move his fingers and toes.

Possible loss of sensation. Test by gently touching the limbs without his knowledge and asking the casualty if he can feel touch or pain.

Even though there is no apparent loss of power or sensation, handle with the utmost care and so prevent a spinal fracture from causing damage to the spinal cord.

Treatment

The aim of first aid here is to prepare the casualty so that he can be moved and transported to the hospital without damaging the spinal cord.

1. Warn the casualty to lie still.
2. If medical aid is readily available:
Do not move the casualty.

Cover him with a blanket and await the arrival of the doctor.

3. If medical aid is not readily available:

Whilst the casualty's shoulders and pelvis are firmly held, place pads of soft material between the thighs, knees and ankles.

Tie the ankles and feet together with a figure-of-eight bandage.

Apply broad bandages round
(i) the thighs
(ii) the knees

Fracture of the ribs

Ribs may be fractured by:

Direct force, if severe. The broken ends of the bone may be driven inwards causing a complicated fracture. The organs most commonly involved are the lungs.

Indirect force, usually produced by pressure on the front and back of the chest, as in crushing. Usually more than one rib is involved.

Signs and symptoms

Sharp pain at the site of the fracture, increased by deep breathing or coughing.

The casualty usually takes short, shallow breaths in an attempt to limit movements and decrease pain.

If internal organs are affected, there may be signs and symptoms of internal bleeding.

There may be an open wound in the chest wall over the fracture, causing a 'sucking wound' of the chest which will lead to asphyxia unless treated immediately.

Treatment

When the fracture is uncomplicated:

1. Support the upper limb on the injured side in an arm sling.

2. Transport as a sitting or walking case unless otherwise indicated.

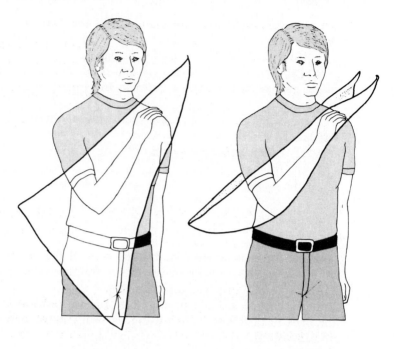

Triangular bandage

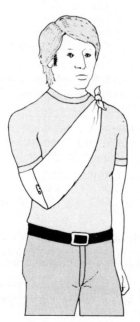

When the fracture is complicated:
1. Any 'sucking wound' must be made airtight immediately.
2. Support the upper limb on the injured side in a triangular sling.
3. Lay the casualty down with head and shoulders raised, and the body inclined towards the injured side.
4. Support the casualty in this position by means of a folded blanket applied lengthwise to his back.
5. Transport to hospital as a stretcher case.

The breastbone

This fracture is usually associated with crush injuries and may be complicated by damage to the underlying chest organs and blood vessels.

Treatment

1. Loosen tight clothing about neck, chest and waist.
2. Place the casualty with his head and shoulders raised, in the most comfortable position, with due regard to associated injuries.
3. Transport as a stretcher case.

Collar-bone

Causes

Indirect force. The usual cause is a fall on the outstretched hand or on the point of the shoulder.
Direct force. The usual cause is a blow.

Treatment

1. Fold two triangular bandages narrow.
2. Pass each narrow bandage through one armpit, encircle the same shoulder and tie behind in a reef knot.
3. Carry the free ends across the back over a pad placed between the shoulder blades; tie opposite ends together, or secure with a third bandage.
As the knots are carefully tightened the shoulders are braced well back, in order to correct the overriding of the broken ends of the clavicle.

4. Support the arm on the injured side in a triangular arm sling.

Shoulder-blade

This rare injury is the result of direct force.

Treatment

1. Remove overcoat and braces (if worn).
2. Place a pad in the armpit.
3. Support the upper limb in a triangular sling, with finger-tips to opposite shoulder.
4. Give further support by securing the upper limb to the chest by a broad bandage applied over the sling.

The upper limb

Upper arm: may occur anywhere along the bone (humerus) and be near or even involve the elbow joint.

Forearm: May involve either the radius or ulna or both, and also the elbow joint.

Treatment

If elbow is not involved:

1. Place the forearm across the chest, finger tips touching the fold of the opposite armpit.
2. Ensure adequate soft padding between the limb and the chest.
3. Support the limb in an arm sling.

Wrist and lower end of forearm

When the lower end of the radius is fractured (Colles's fracture) there may or may not be considerable deformity present. It is a common fracture and can be mistaken for a sprain of the wrist.

Treatment

1. Protect the forearm and wrist by placing it on a fold of soft padding.
2. Support the limb in an arm sling.

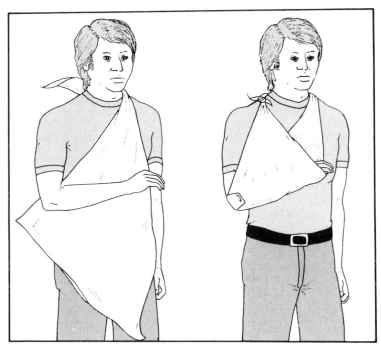

Arm sling

3. Give further support by securing the upper limb to the chest by a broad bandage applied over the sling.

Knee-cap (patella)

A fracture may be the result of muscular action which causes the bone to snap in two. It may also be fractured by direct force.

Treatment

1. Lay the casualty on his back with head and shoulders raised and supported (semi-recumbent position).
2. Raise and support the injured limb in a comfortable position.
3. Apply a splint along the back of the limb, reaching from the buttock to beyond the heel.

293

Crushed foot

Commonly caused by a heavy weight dropping on or going over the foot. A fracture should be suspected when there is pain, swelling and loss of power.

Treatment

1. Carefully remove shoe or boot and sock or stocking, cutting if necessary.
2. Treat a wound, if present.
3. Apply a well-padded splint to the sole of the foot, reaching from the heel to the toes.
4. Secure the splint with a figure-of-eight bandage as follows:
Place the centre of a broad bandage on the sole of the foot, cross the ends over the instep and carry to the back of the ankle. Cross them, bring them to the front of the ankle and cross them once more, then pass them under the sole of the foot. Tie off over the splint.
5. Raise and support the foot in a comfortable position.

Heart attacks
These result from a reduction in the blood supply to the muscular wall of the heart.

There are two varieties: (1) angina pectoris (severe pain in the chest); and (2) obstruction of a coronary artery in the wall of the heart.

1. *Angina pectoris*

The channels of the arteries supplying blood to the heart become too narrow for an adequate supply to the heart muscle when it is working harder than normal. Excitement or over-exertion brings on an attack of pain in the chest which often spreads to the left shoulder and arm and to the fingers. The pain may also spread to the throat and jaws and to the other upper limb. It is relieved by rest and usually lasts only a few minutes.

2. *Coronary Obstruction*

The blood clots suddenly in a coronary artery and blocks it. The onset of pain is not necessarily related to exertion. The casualty is gripped by an excruciating vice-like pain behind the breast-bone; it may radiate into the upper limbs, throat or jaw. Rest is essential, but may not ease the pain.

Signs and symptoms

In angina pectoris and coronary obstruction the patient suffers severely from shock.

Severe pain may force him to stop what he is doing and sit down or lean against a wall for support.

He may feel giddy and sink to the ground. Even when shock is slight the patient may still be seriously ill as a further severe attack may follow.

He is often short of breath.

He may become unconscious.

The pulse is weak and may be irregular.

Note: In coronary obstruction death may result from the stopping of the heart beat.

Treatment

The aim of first aid in cases of acute heart attack is to reduce the work of the heart and sustain the patient during an attack.

1. *Do not* move the patient unnecessarily, but place him in the most comfortable position. This is usually:
– Semi-recumbent, with head and shoulders raised on two or more pillows; or
– Supported in a sitting position if this makes his breathing easier.
2. Loosen clothing about neck, chest and waist.
3. If breathing fails, begin artificial respiration immediately and, if necessary, give external heart compression. Both these procedures may have to be continued on the way to hospital.
4. Arrange for urgent transport to hospital, obtaining medical aid if available. Administration of oxygen may be required.

Note: people liable to heart pain (angina) often carry tablets (glyceril trinitrate) which are useful for the prevention of an attack when one is felt coming on.

Congestive heart failure

During chronic heart disease, heart failure and collapse may occur. The condition is different from coronary obstruction. It resembles that of an acute heart attack, but the patient may be cyanosed and may cough up large amounts of blood-stained sputum.

Treatment

As for acute heart attack, but support the patient in a sitting position. Do not lay him flat as he will not be able to get sufficient air into his lungs and may become asphyxiated. Be prepared to deal with vomiting and bowel action.

Heat exhaustion

The onset of heat exhaustion is slow and gives rise to a shocked condition due to a salt and water deficiency.

Causes

Exposure to excessive heat, especially moist heat. Is commonly found in newcomers to very hot climates. Fluid and salt loss is considerable from excessive sweating and is often aggravated further by a gastrointestinal upset with diarrhoea and vomiting.

A person who is acclimatized to the tropics may also be affected by water deficiency following a severe attack of malaria or other tropical fever.

Signs and symptoms

Muscular cramp from salt deficiency is an early sign.

The casualty is exhausted and may be restless.

The face is pale and cold and has a clammy sweat; there may be sudden collapse and loss of consciousness.

Pulse and breathing are rapid.

Temperature may be normal, sub-normal, or slightly elevated.

A complaint of headache, dizziness and nausea, and sometimes of abdominal cramp may be made.

Sudden movement may cause fainting (syncope).

Treatment

1. Place and keep the casualty in cool surroundings.
2. If conscious, give cold water to drink. If casualty has had excessive sweating, cramps, diarrhoea and/or vomiting, add half a teaspoonful of common salt to each pint (half a litre) of water.
3. Obtain medical aid.

Heat stroke

The onset is more sudden and may be preceded by heat exhaustion.

Causes

Heat stroke may be brought on by a high atmospheric temperature, with a hot, drying wind, or by a high humidity and lack of air current. It may also be caused by malaria or other debilitating illness. The body can no longer control its temperature by sweating.

Signs and symptoms

Unconsciousness may come on quickly. A temperature of 40°C (104°F) or more may occur.

The casualty is restless, and, if conscious, complains of headache, dizziness and feeling hot.

The face is flushed, the skin hot and dry to the touch.

The pulse is full and bounding.

Breathing is noisy.

There may be confusion or stupor; coma may result.

Treatment

The aim of first aid here is to reduce the casualty's temperature as quickly as possible.

1. Strip the casualty and wrap in a wet, cold sheet; keep it wet until his temperature has been lowered to 38°C (101°F).
2. Place him in the recovery position.
3. Direct currents of air on to him from above and below by hand or by electric fans.
4. On recovery, the casualty, with a dry sheet over him, should be transported to air-conditioned accommodation to prevent relapse.
5. If his temperature rises again, repeat the treatment.
6. Send to hospital.

Hiccups

Commonly the result of a digestive disturbance or 'nervousness'. Relief may be obtained in various ways, e.g. sips of water, holding the breath or distracting the attention.

If the condition persists for more than a few hours, the person's doctor should be informed.

Hypothermia

This is a dangerous lowering of the body temperature. It may occur at any age, but babies and the elderly who lack the ability to regulate their own temperature, even when not fatigued, are most at risk. A loss of surface heat is followed by cooling of the deep tissues and organs of the body.

Causes

Exposure to cold – from weather or in an unheated home.

Prolonged immersion in cold water e.g. shipwreck in Arctic or Antarctic conditions.

Lowering of sensibility to cold by alcohol, drugs or poisoning.

A contributory cause may be a medical condition, e.g. diabetes.

Infants. Babies must be kept constantly warm during the first few weeks of life as they cannot regulate their own body temperature.

Elderly and infirm. Those living alone, especially pensioners on an inadequate diet, may be found in a state of stupor on the floor, collapsed in an outside passage, or lying unconscious in bed. In such cases, they may be fully clothed. This condition can easily be mistaken for a 'stroke' or heart attack.

Signs and symptoms

Infants are quiet and refuse food. Pink face, hands and feet, if present, are deceptive.

The elderly and infirm are pale and in a state of collapse. The casualty is deathly cold to the touch.

The pulse is slow, weak or imperceptible.

Breathing is slow and shallow.

Treatment

The aim of first aid in all these cases is to prevent further heat loss, improve body heat and circulation, to obtain medical aid, or transport the casualty to hospital.

1. Place the casualty between blankets so that the body temperature can recover gradually.

2. If conscious, give tepid or warm, sweet drinks. Do not use hot water bottles or electric blankets as this will cause sudden dilation of the superficial blood vessels, taking away blood from the deep tissues and essential organs. This may cause a fatal collapse due to a drop in the casualty's blood pressure and temperature.

Poisonings

A poison is any substance – solid, liquid or gas – which, when taken into the body in sufficient amounts, may damage health or even destroy life.

It may be taken either accidentally or intentionally:

1. Through the lungs – breathing poisonous gases or fumes.

2. By the mouth – swallowing.

3. By injection – under the skin.

4. By absorption – through the skin.

Through the lungs

This occurs mainly by breathing household gas fumes from fires, stoves, motor exhausts, or smoke. Poisoning from industrial gases may also occur, e.g. carbon tetrachloride (contained in some fire extinguishers and dry cleaning solvents). Trichorethylene (present in de-greasing and dry cleaning agents).

By the mouth

Swallowed poisons act quickly, either:

1. Directly on the food passage causing retching, vomiting, pain and often diarrhoea. Common causes are poisonous berries (see page 244) and infected and decomposed food. Severe symptoms are caused by corrosives (strong acids and alkalis) which burn the lips, mouth, gullet and stomach and cause intense pain, or
2. On the nervous system after absorption into the blood.

Common causes are excessive alcohol, tablets and solutions taken to relieve pain (aspirin, preparations containing opium derivatives) or to produce sleep (barbiturate drugs). A few poisons act on the nervous system causing delirium (e.g. belladonna) or fits (e.g. strychnine, prussic acid).

By injection under the skin

These arise from bites of poisonous reptiles, some animals and certain insects, or by hypodermic syringe, e.g. deliberate taking of drugs, such as heroin.

By absorption through the skin

Common causes are certain pesticides used by farmers (such as parathion, malathion etc.). They cause convulsions if swallowed.

Warning: Leaving aside the possibility of death, life may be endangered by:

Asphyxia, which may occur from the results of poisons,

especially those taken through the lungs or acting on the nervous system.

Convulsions, which may occur as a result of poisons absorbed through the skin.

Coma, which may occur from the results of the poisons in any group.

General rules for treatment of poisoning

The aim of first aid is to sustain life by diluting the poisons and removing urgently to hospital.

1. If the casualty is conscious:

Ask him quickly what happened. Remember he may lose consciousness at any time.

2. If there are no signs of burns on the lips or mouth from corrosive acids or alkalis, make him vomit repeatedly by:

Tickling the back of his throat with your fingers.

3. If lips and mouth show signs of burns do not induce vomiting but dilute the poison by giving quantities of water, milk or barley water.

Remove the casualty to hospital quickly by car or ambulance.

4. If the casualty is unconscious:

If breathing freely, place him in the recovery position, thus ensuring an open airway.

If breathing is failing or has ceased, commence artificial respiration immediately. This may have to be continued until hospital treatment can be given, as part of the breathing mechanism has been disturbed by the poison.

Remove the casualty to hospital quickly by ambulance.

5. Send any particulars of the suspected cause, if known, to hospital with the casualty, together with:

Any remaining poison.

Any box, carton, bottle or other container which may help to identify the poison.

Any vomited matter.

Note: Suicides often take all the tablets and dispose of the containers.

Additional treatment for special cases of poisoning

Pesticides

The casualty must not be allowed to exert himself at all.
1. Remove contaminated clothing.
2. If convulsions are present, treat as a fit.
3. Sponge head, back of neck, spine and body freely with cold water.
4. Place casualty in a current of air. If necessary, fan him.
5. Give casualty as much water or well-sweetened drink as he can swallow.

Rat poison

These food baits are highly poisonous and dangerous to children.

1. Induce vomiting.
2. Send to hospital any child who has eaten these baits.

Rupture (abdominal hernia)

This condition is a protrusion of some part of the abdominal contents through the muscular wall of the abdomen under the skin.

It occurs most frequently in the groin, but it is not uncommon at the navel or through the scar of an abdominal operation. It may occur after exercise, whilst lifting heavy objects, coughing or even when straining on the lavatory when constipated.

The condition may arise as painless swelling, which may persist or worsen. It may occur suddenly with swelling, pain and possibly vomiting.

'Strangulated' hernia, an urgent surgical problem, may present these symptoms and signs.

Treatment

1. Reassure the casualty.
2. Lay him down and support his head and shoulders, bend and support his knees; if vomiting occurs, or seems likely, place him in the recovery position.

3. Seek medical aid if pain or vomiting persists.
Do not attempt to reduce the swelling.

Sprain

A sprain occurs at a joint and is caused by the wrenching or tearing of the ligaments and tissues connected with the joint.

Signs and symptoms

Pain at the joint.
Swelling about the joint and later bruising.
Inability to use the joint without increasing the pain.

Treatment

1. Rest and support the joint in the most comfortable position for the casualty.
2. Carefully expose the joint.
3. Apply pressure over the joint by surrounding it with a good layer of cotton wool, keeping it in position by a firmly tied bandage; or apply a cold compress to the joint.

If a sprain of the ankle occurs out-of-doors, do not remove the boot or shoe but give additional support by applying a figure-of-eight bandage over the boot or shoe.

Note: In all doubtful cases treat as a fracture.

Stings (Bees, Hornets, Wasps)

Treatment

1. Remove the sting, if present, using the point of a needle which has been sterilized by passing it through a flame and then cooling it.
2. Antihistamine creams are useful if applied immediately. Otherwise, apply surgical spirit, a weak ammonia solution, or a solution of bicarbonate of soda.
3. If the sting is in the mouth, give a mouthwash of one teaspoonful (5 ml) of bicarbonate of soda to a tumbler of water. If there is much swelling in the mouth or difficulty

in breathing, place the casualty in the recovery position and give him ice to suck. Seek medical aid immediately.

Strain

A strain is the over-stretching of a muscle.

Signs and symptoms

Sudden sharp pain at the site of injury. In the case of a limb, the muscle may swell and cause severe cramp.

Treatment

1. Place the casualty in the most comfortable position.
2. Steady and support the injured part.
3. Arrange for medical aid.

Sunburn

Direct exposure of the skin to the sun's rays may produce itching, burning and redness, due to the dilatation of the blood vessels in the skin, or even superficial burns of the unacclimatized skin before a protective tan has developed. It can also be caused by sun-bathing with the body wet with sea water or sweat.

It may also arise in conditions of ice or snow or of desert sand, when the severity is increased by the reflection of ultra-violet radiations from these surfaces.

If the heat has been excessive, swelling and blistering may occur even after a short exposure. The head should be protected to prevent heat stroke.

Prevention of sunburn is by very gradual exposure of the skin to the sun in order to obtain a tan. In severe conditions, not more than five minutes' exposure on the first day is recommended.

Treatment

1. Rest in the shade.
2. Give a cold drink.

3. If sunburn is severe, seek medical aid.
Immersion of the part in cool water may have a soothing effect.

Note: Various skin lotions and creams are available for slight irritations or redness of the skin.

Stroke – see apoplexy.

Shock

Shock is a condition resulting from a lessening of the activities of the vital functions of the body arising from a lack of blood supply. It may accompany injuries, severe pain or sudden illness. The severity of shock depends upon the nature and extent of the injury or other cause and may vary from a feeling of faintness even to death. It is associated with many conditions and injuries.

Causes

Severe bleeding:
    External – e.g. from an artery or ruptured varicose vein.
    Internal – e.g. into the abdomen, the chest cavity of the tissues surrounding the broken bone of a limb.
Burns.
Crush injuries.
Heart failure.
Acute heart attack.
Acute abdominal emergencies.
Perforation of the stomach, ruptured appendix.
Loss of body fluid.
Recurrent vomiting and severe diarrhoea.

Signs and symptoms

Casualty will become extremely pale:
    His skin will become cold and clammy, with profuse sweating.
    He may feel faint or giddy or have blurring of vision.
    He may feel sick and may vomit.

He may complain of thirst.

He may be very anxious.

His consciousness may be clouded.

His pulse increases in rate; tending to become weak and thready.

His breathing is shallow and rapid.

Treatment

1. Lay casualty down and deal with the injury or under-lying cause of the shock.

2. Waste no time. Get the casualty to hospital. His life may depend upon immediate blood transfusion and other hospital treatment.

3. Keep his head low and turned to one side with the lower limbs raised, when possible.

If there is an injury to the head, chest or abdomen, the shoulders should be raised slightly and supported, with the head turned to one side.

If vomiting seems likely, or if the casualty is unconscious, place him carefully in the recovery position.

4. Loosen clothing at the neck, chest and waist.

5. If the casualty complains of thirst, moisten his lips with water.

6. Protect him when necessary with a blanket or sheet.

7. Keep frequent records of the pulse and respiration rates if removal to hospital is likely to be delayed.

Do not heat the casualty or use hot water bottles, as this draws blood from the vital organs to the skin.

Do not give the casualty anything to drink.

Do not move him unnecessarily. Leaving the casualty in the position in which he is found frequently outweighs the benefits of any other action. The more serious the injury, the more important it is not to move the casualty more than is necessary.

'Winding'

The result of a blow in the upper part of the abdomen (solar plexus) which may cause fainting or even collapse.

Treatment

1. Place the casualty in the recovery position.
2. Loosen tight clothing at the neck, chest and waist.
3. Gently massage the upper abdomen.

Section Four

20. Brief Guide to the re-organized National Health Service

General

The National Health Service Act of 1946 aimed at promoting 'the establishment in England and Wales of a comprehensive health service, designed to secure improvement in the physical and mental health of the people of England and Wales and the prevention, diagnosis and treatment of illness'. Through the Act the Minister of Health was made responsible to Parliament for seeing that health services of every kind, and of the highest possible quality, were available to everyone who needed them. The NHS (Scotland) Act 1947, laid similar responsibilities on the Secretary of State for Scotland. Both these Acts were passed by Parliament and came into force on 5 July 1948.

Under the National Health Service, the essential freedoms have been safeguarded, for the public is free to use the service or not as he pleases. The patient can choose his family doctor, and, if he wishes, change to another. The doctor is free from interference in his clinical judgment, and may accept private patients whilst playing a part in the NHS. The service is available free to all residents in Britain according to their medical need, except that certain small charges are made for some items. Treatment can be given under the emergency provisions of the service to any visitor from abroad who falls ill during his visit, but those who come to Britain specifically for treatment are expected to pay for it. About 97 per cent of the population of Britain are using the service.

Organization in England

From 1948 to 1974, the NHS was administered in three parts – the hospital and specialist services, the general practitioner services and the local authority services. Under the NHS Reorganization Act of 1973 these services were unified, with just over 100 regional and area health authorities taking control in place of over 600 boards, committees and councils that had previously been responsible for them.

The new arrangements came into force on 1 April 1974, and provide for three levels of planning: central strategic planning and monitoring by the Department of Health and Social Security; regional planning and general supervision of operation by regional health authorities (RHAs); and area planning and operational control by area health authorities (AHAs).

The Department of Health and Social Security (DHSS)

The DHSS came into being on 1 November 1968, as an amalgamation of the Ministry of Health (first established in 1919) and the Ministry of Social Security. The section dealing with health has a staff of about 5,000 people, and is mainly a central supervisory department for the general organization, planning and financing of the health and welfare services. The Secretary of State for Social Services is the head of the DHSS. This is a political appointment, as are those of the Minister of State, the Parliamentary Under-Secretary of State (Health) and the Parliamentary Under-Secretary of State (Social Security). The two senior permanent officials of the DHSS are the Permanent Secretary and the Chief Medical Officer: they are both members of the Civil Service, as are the rest of the staff of the DHSS. But none of the staff employed by regional and area authorities in the NHS are civil servants.

The Secretary of State is responsible to Parliament for the NHS and the role of the DHSS is to assist him by:

(a) Settling the kind, scale and balance of service to be provided in regions and areas.

(b) Guiding, supporting and (to the extent that this is desirable) controlling RHAs. Here it is the Department's job to help the authorities to understand the guide-lines and the reasoning behind them. It also allocates to the RHAs the necessary resources.

(c) Obtaining or developing resources which strongly influence the adequacy, efficiency and economy of the services. This requires specialist work on particular resources – personnel, finance, property and building, supply. The Department has a special responsibility in relation to staffing – for instance, forecasting staff requirements, planning the number of training places, etc.

(d) Carrying out other functions which are best organized centrally, such as some types of research, standardization and preparation of national statistics.

(e) Supporting the Secretary of State in his Parliamentary and public duties.

Regional Health Authorities

There are 14 Regional Health Authorities (RHAs) in England each consisting of between three and eleven health areas. The RHA forms part of the chain of responsibility running from the Secretary of State to each AHA. The Chairman and members of the RHA are appointed by the Secretary of State after consultations with interested organizations, including the universities, the main local authorities, the main health professions and the TUC. Members are unpaid (but entitled to travelling and other allowances) but the Chairman may be paid on a part-time basis.

The role of the RHA is to develop strategic plans and priorities based on a review of the needs identified by the AHAs. It is responsible for allocating resources among AHAs, agreeing area plans with them and monitoring their performance. The most important of the RHAs' executive functions is the design and construction of new hospitals and other health buildings. It is also responsible for identifying, in consultation with the AHAs, services which need a regional rather than an area approach and arranging for their provision.

Area Health Authorities

There are ninety Area Health Authorities (AHAs) in England whose boundaries generally match those of the new non-metropolitan counties and metropolitan districts of local government. In London the health authority boundaries correspond to those of an individual London Borough in four cases, and two, three, or in one case, four London Boroughs grouped together in the remaining twelve cases. The AHA is the operational NHS authority, responsible for assessing needs in its area and for planning, organizing and administering area health services to meet them. It employs the staff who work at area headquarters and in the districts. It is also responsible for services such as catering and domestic, as well as for other supportive services which back up the health professions and, in so doing, contribute to patient care.

The Chairman of the AHA is appointed by the Secretary of State after consultation with the Chairman of the RHA. There are about fifteen members for each AHA, four of whom are appointed by the corresponding local authority, one by the university concerned (areas with substantial teaching facilities are administered by AHA (Teaching), and the remaining members appointed by the RHA after consultation with the main health professions, the trade unions and other organizations. An AHA always includes doctors and at least one nurse or midwife, but otherwise the proportion of professional members is not laid down. Members are unpaid (but entitled to travelling and other allowances) but the Chairman may be paid on a part-time basis.

Health Districts

The day-to-day running of the services for which each AHA is responsible is based on health districts. These always contain a district general hospital and usually have a population of between 150,000 and 300,000. The AHA's decide the number of districts in their areas and these vary between one and six. There is no statutory authority at district level, as there is at area or regional level, and responsibility for the day-to-day operation of the services at district level lies with the district management team of about six senior medical, nursing, administrative and finance officers.

At district level there are also health care planning teams whose function is to determine health care needs of groups of patients (e.g. elderly, mentally ill, mentally handicapped children, etc.) or to look at particular problems (e.g. review of primary care services, re-organization of out-patient department, etc.).

Social Services

Under the new arrangements, as under the old, health service costs are met mainly through central government funds from tax revenue. Social services, on the other hand, are planned and controlled by local government authorities (sharing, in most cases, the same boundaries as area health authorities), and their costs are met mainly through local government funds. Although separately financed it is very important that health and social services should be planned jointly, particularly for the old, the mentally ill and mentally handicapped. There is, therefore, under the 1973 Act a statutory responsibility for all health authorities to collaborate in planning with their corresponding local government authorities. Co-operation in this field is vital to the success of the re-organized NHS.

Community Health Councils

A completely new feature of the reorganized NHS is the establishment of Community Health Councils (CHCs). These CHCs represent the views of the consumer. There is one for each area of a health district. Half the members of the Council are appointed by the local authorities of which the area, or part of it, is included in the CHC's district; at least one-third by voluntary bodies concerned locally with the NHS, and the remainder by RHA after consultation with other organizations. The number of members varies according to local circumstances, but there are usually between twenty and thirty. Members are unpaid, but entitled to travelling and other expenses. Councils appoint their own Chairmen from among their members.

The Council's basic job is to represent to the AHA the interests of the public in the health service in its district. Councils have powers to secure information, to visit hospitals and other institutions, and have access to the AHA and in particular to its senior officers administering the district services. Councils may bring to the notice of the AHA potential causes of local complaint, but their function is distinct from that of the AHAs' complaints machinery and of the Health Service Commissioner.

The AHA is required to consult the Council(s) on its plans for health service developments – e.g. closures of hospitals or departments of hospitals, or their change of use. The full AHA meets representatives of all its Councils at least once a year. The Council publishes an annual report (and may publish other reports) and the AHA is required to publish replies recording action taken on the issues raised.

Health Service Commissioner

Another new feature of the NHS is the appointment of a Health Service Commissioner to investigate complaints against the NHS authorities. This is an important extension of the ombudsman principle in the public service. The necessary legislation is part of the NHS Reorganization Act, and since 1 April, 1974 his jurisdiction has covered the whole of the unified NHS. He does not, however, investigate complaints which, in his opinion, relate to the exercise of clinical judgement by doctors and other staff, nor does he deal with complaints for which statutory procedures already exist (e.g. those about general medical and dental practitioners, pharmacists and opticians, which continue to be dealt with under the service committee procedure) or which he thinks the complainant could reasonably pursue through the courts of law.

The complainant has direct access to the Commissioner, who, however, does not investigate a complaint until he is satisfied that the health authority concerned has had a reasonable opportunity to investigate it and reply to the complainant who, despite this, is still dissatisfied. Complaints to the Commissioner do not have to be made by the patient himself: there are some instances where the patient is unable to act for himself, and in such cases the complaint may be made on his behalf.

Voluntary Services

Under the new arrangements voluntary bodies, which have always played an important part in the development of the health and welfare services, are being encouraged, in close co-operation with the area health and local authorities, to increase and extend their activities. Through their membership of the Community Health Councils they are able to influence the way in which the health services are developed. The recent growth in the number of organizers co-ordinating voluntary help in hospitals will continue, and this method of co-ordination is being extended to the wider field of voluntary work in the community.

The RHAs and AHAs will be able to make grants in support of voluntary bodies which provide and promote services within the general scope of the authorities' responsibilities. Financial help for national activities continues to come from the central Department. As all this voluntary activity develops, it is important to emphasize that the role of volunteers is no longer seen as being to plug gaps in the welfare state, but rather to complement and enrich the quality of life for people in need, whether they are living in their own homes, in hospital or in any form of residential care. It is also to pioneer new ideas and to develop in the hospital and its neighbourhood a real sense of community involvement in the services which, as taxpayers or rate-payers, they largely finance.

21 A Guide to other available help

Aegis (Aid for the Elderly in Government Institutions)
10, Hampstead Grove, London, NW3 Tel no: 01 435 6155.
Aegis was formed in 1965 to protect the interests of elderly patients in Government Institutions. It has three basic aims: to call public attention to some serious defects that exist in the care of these patients; to devise remedies for such defects; and to propagate modern methods of geriatric care with strong emphasis on rehabilitation.

Age Concern
Bernard Sunley House, 60 Pitcairn Road, Mitcham, Surrey. Tel no: 640 5431.
Age Concern is an independent national charity bringing together in consultation voluntary societies, government departments, individuals with special experience in the care of the elderly and representatives of old people's welfare committees. It exists to co-ordinate statutory and voluntary services for the elderly and to represent nationally the needs and views of old people. It publishes a quarterly magazine, handbooks and leaflets on aspects of the care of old people.

Al-Anon Family Groups, United Kingdom and Eire
c/o St Giles Centre, Camberwell Church Street, London, SE5 8RB Tel no: 01 703 0397.
Al-Anon is a fellowship of relatives and friends of alcoholics who share their experiences, strength and hope with each other in order to solve the problem of living with the alcoholic. Members have demonstrated that changed family attitudes can bring about recovery. The office is open from 10 am to 4 pm daily, Mondays to Fridays.

Association for All Speech Impaired Children
Room 11, Nuffield Hearing and Speech Centre, Swinton Street, London, WC1. Tel. no 01 837 8855.
The Association for All Speech Impaired Children was started in 1967 by professional people concerned with the

315

plight of children with severe disorders of speech and language and with the distress of their parents. The Association's first Executive Committee consisted of parents, teachers and doctors. Its aims are:

1. To sponsor and support education in the nature of normal development in speech, and in how to detect and help children with difficulties of speech and language.
2. To provide an advisory service for parents and others; to co-ordinate the work of existing organizations, and health, educational and speech therapy services.
3. To promote the study of normal development in speech in infancy and the training of teachers.
4. To sponsor and support research into assessment and diagnosis of and suitable treatment for, children with difficulties of speech and language.

Association for Spina Bifida and Hydrocephalus
30, Devonshire Street, London, W1N 2EB Tel no: 01 486 6100 or 01 935 9060.

The Association for Spina Bifida and Hydrocephalus was formed in 1966 and has seventy local Associations in England, Wales and Northern Ireland, and a sister Association in Scotland. The Association has the twin aims of supporting and helping those with these conditions and their families, and of promoting and sponsoring research into treatment and causes. The Association publishes a quarterly magazine, *Link*, and a number of other publications which are widely used in this country and overseas.

Bath Association for the Study of Dyslexia
18, The Circus, Bath, Somerset, BA1 2ET
Tel no: Bath 28880.

The object of the Bath Association for the Study of Dyslexia is to establish the incidence and extent of specific language disability (dyslexia) in children and adults and to provide remedial treatment either as an advisory body or by tuition, and to assist in the distribution of knowledge to teachers.

316

BREAK (Holidays for Handicapped and Deprived Children)
*100, First Avenue, Bush Hill Park, Enfield, Middlesex
Tel no: 01 366 0253.*
BREAK provides holidays throughout the year at its
centre, The Sandcastle, Hunstanton, Norfolk. Children are
accepted up to 15 years of age. Older children are considered
according to circumstances. Deprived, disturbed, maladjusted children, as well as all kinds of physically and mentally
handicapped children, are taken. Brothers and sisters of
children in need are welcome where it is considered undesirable to separate them. It is occasionally possible to
accommodate entire families or a handicapped parent with
the children.

The British Association of the Hard of Hearing
Briarfield, Syke Ings, Iver, Bucks.
The British Association of the Hard of Hearing offers
assistance with all problems arising from loss of hearing
total or partial, to people with normal speech and education,
on lip-reading, hearing aids, social life and employment. The
Association has over 200 social clubs throughout the
United Kingdom. It arranges educational week-end courses
and holidays. All workers are voluntary and nearly all are
of impaired hearing.

British Council for Rehabilitation of the Disabled
*Tavistock House (South), Tavistock Square, London,
WC1H 9LB Tel no: 01 387 4037/8.*
The British Council for Rehabilitation of the Disabled
was founded in 1944 to assess the needs of the disabled and
to develop a comprehensive rehabilitation service. The
Council arranges educational courses and conferences on
rehabilitation and on problems of disease and disablement,
with particular reference to employment. It also disseminates
information on a wide range of subjects and, through its
preparatory training bureau, arranges correspondence courses
and personal tuition for long-stay patients in hospitals,
sanatoria and at home. The Council has an engineering
department concerned with aids to mobility. It publishes a
quarterly journal, *Rehabilitation*. The Council founded and
sponsors the Association of Disabled Professionals.

British Diabetic Association
3–6, Alfred Place, London, WC1E 7EE Tel no: 01 636 7355.

The object of the British Diabetic Association is to help the diabetic to understand his condition and its treatment so that he can live a full and useful life. It raises money for research, provides an advisory service on any diabetic problem, apart from medical, and publishes *Balance* every two months. There are 120 branches throughout the United Kingdom. There is a Professional Services Section for persons with professional qualifications, intended principally for those in the professions supplementary to medicine. Meetings are held in April and September. A Medical and Scientific Section aims to promote the study of the causes and treatment of diabetes and associated diseases and to help to diffuse among doctors and scientific workers knowledge of the scientific and clinical aspects of diabetes.

British Epilepsy Association (Epilepsy Information Unit)
3–6, Alfred Place, London, WC1E 7EE. Tel no: 01 580 2704.

As the main problem of epilepsy is lack of understanding, the British Epilepsy Association was formed to educate and inform the public about this condition. Modern methods of diagnosis and treatment can control epilepsy but, after diagnosis, the patient and his family are confronted with various problems such as education, employment, marriage, whether or not to have children. The Association can supply information and literature on these problems and runs a personal advice service. A wide range of conferences, courses and symposia are arranged for professional groups, and lecturers are available on request.

British Guild for Sudden Infant Death Study
28, Ty Gwen Crescent, Penylan, Cardiff, Wales
Tel no: Cardiff 35252.

The Guild has been founded to stimulate public awareness of the sudden infant death syndrome ('cot death') and, particularly, to emphasize its natural, non-accidental nature. The objects are to stimulate research, bring about administrative reforms in registration and coroner's procedures and contact newly bereaved parents, offering them sympathy and information, and relieving the almost universal feelings of self reproach.

British Migraine Association
Evergreen, Ottermeade Lane, Ottershaw, Chertsey
Tel no: 093 28 73242.

The British Migraine Association exists for the encouragement of migraine sufferers, to support research into the causes and alleviation of migraine, to present the patient's views and interests, to offer a friendly and helpful service to all sufferers, to stimulate medical interest and to keep all members informed of progress in research by means of a quarterly newsletter.

The British Polio Fellowship
Bell Close, West End Road, Ruislip, Middlesex, HA4 6LP
Tel no: Ruislip 75515/16/17.

The British Polio Fellowship, registered as a charity as the Infantile Paralysis Fellowship, is the national voluntary organization for those disabled by poliomyelitis. There are eighty-three branches throughout the United Kingdom. Its objects are to foster the fellowship of people who have had poliomyelitis; to find means of training members to be self-supporting; to alleviate loneliness and to bring those who need advice or assistance into contact with available sources of help. It provides a personal welfare service and runs holiday hotels, residential homes and schemes for sheltered work.

British Red Cross Society
9, Grosvenor Crescent, London, SW1X 7EJ
Tel no: 01 235 5454.

The objects of the British Red Cross Society include the improvement of health, the prevention of disease, and the mitigation of suffering. The Society trains its members in first aid, auxiliary nursing and welfare to provide regular nursing support to hospitals and supplement the domiciliary care of the sick, particularly in time of emergency. Other activities include assistance at blood donor sessions and escorting patients on journeys. In hospitals, it runs a service of trolley shops and canteens, telephone trolleys, books and picture libraries, beauty care, language cards and, on occasion, interpreters for foreign patients, visiting those far from home, preparation for patients' admission and discharge and the care of relatives of the dangerously ill. It lends medical equipment and helps in clinics and health centres throughout the country.

The Junior Red Cross is formed of children from five to sixteen years old, who are given practical training in primary health, first aid, home nursing, hygiene, infant and child care, prevention of accidents, protection against fire, drill, rescue and messenger work. They help the sick and suffering in the many Red Cross services suited to their age, especially helping physically handicapped children and the elderly. They co-operate with junior members in other countries at International Study Centres and Exhibitions, send parcels of 'self-help' gifts such as First Aid Training Kits through their Gift Scheme to the Society's branches overseas, and provide knitted blankets and Relief Kits for children in disaster areas.

British Society for Music Therapy
48, Lanchester Road, London, N6 4TA Tel no: 01 883 1331.
The object of the British Society for Music Therapy is to promote the use of music therapy in the treatment, education, rehabilitation and training of children and adults suffering from physical, mental or emotional disorder. The Society publishes the *British Journal of Music Therapy* and a number of pamphlets. It organizes meetings and conferences which are open to the general public. It offers a one-year post-graduate course leading to the Diploma in Music Therapy in association with the Guildhall School of Music and Drama. The membership includes medical practitioners, psychologists, educationalists, social workers, therapists, musicians and various organizations concerned with the welfare of handicapped adults and children.

Cancer Information Association
Gloucester Green, Oxford, OX1 2EQ
Tel no: Oxford 46654.
The objects of the Cancer Information Association are to alleviate the fear of cancer among the public and to encourage the recognition of early warning signs which could indicate cancer and the seeking of medical advice, which can lead to early treatment. The Association provides lectures

and film programmes to any organization upon request, and supplies a list of publications on cancer education.

Cancer Research Campaign
2 Carlton House Terrace, London, SW1Y 5AR
Tel no: 01 930 8972.

The Cancer Research Campaign exists to attack and defeat the disease of cancer in all its forms and to promote its cure by research into its causes and treatments. It is supported entirely by voluntary contributions. It makes grants (in response to applications and on the recommendation of its scientific committee) for cancer research at appropriate universities, hospitals and institutions throughout the United Kingdom, to certain British Commonwealth territories overseas, and for projects by suitably qualified individuals.

The Children's Research Fund
6, Castle Street, Liverpool, L2 0NA
Tel no: Liverpool 236 2844.

The Children's Research Fund exists to finance research into all children's diseases and child health problems at child health research centres and university departments of child health in the United Kingdom, and supplies the Dahl Wade valve for the treatment of hydrocephalus at cost to most countries throughout the world.

The Coeliac Society of Great Britain and Northern Ireland
PO Box 181, London, NW2 2QY.

The Coeliac Society is a voluntary organization which exists to promote the welfare of adults and children with this condition. The Society is open to any medically diagnosed coeliac, and information is also supplied to any member of the medical and allied professions whose work brings him into contact with coeliacs. The Society has published *The Coeliac Handbook* (for Coeliacs), *The Coeliac Condition* (for medical workers). A film, *On the Coeliac Affliction*, is available, on loan, from Concord Films Council Limited, Nacton, Ipswich, Suffolk.

321

Colostomy Welfare Group
38–39, Eccleston Square, London, SW1V 1PB
Tel no: 01 828 5175.

The Colostomy Welfare Group provides a welfare service for patients throughout Great Britain and Northern Ireland who have had, or are about to undergo, colostomy operations. The Group strives to facilitate mental and physical adjustment by allaying fear and anxiety and by teaching and helping patients to adapt themselves to a new way of life. This service is available to hospitals, local health authorities, district nursing associations and individual patients free of charge.

Community Relations Commission
15–16, Bedford Street, London, WC2E 9HX
Tel no: 01 240 1051.

The Community Relations Commission is a statutory body established under the Race Relations Act 1968 to help people of different races and cultures to live and work together in harmony. It advises the Home Secretary on matters of community relations, and co-ordinates and helps finance the work of voluntary local community relations councils of which there are seventy-nine throughout Britain. It employs specialist officers to advise on education, youth, health and welfare in a multi-racial society and publishes material on these topics. Conferences and seminars are organized for a range of professional groups, including health and social workers, teachers, youth leaders and police.

Community Service Volunteers
237, Pentonville Road, London, N1 9NJ Tel no: 01 278 6601.

Community Service Volunteers involves young people in situations of human need throughout the British Isles. Each year over 2000 volunteers give full-time service for any time from four to twelve months in children's homes, borstals, with immigrants, in schools, in homes and centres for the elderly, or with the physically and mentally handicapped, in return only for their board, lodging and pocket money. Many work in hospitals, often on the wards, sometimes involving local volunteers. Over 1000 schools and colleges subscribe to the Advisory Service, School and Community Kits (SACK); CSV also offers a special Advisory Service to hospitals, exploring ways of involving volunteers either from the local community, full-time, or through work camps.

Consumers' Association

14 Buckingham Street, London, WC2 Tel no: 01 839 1222.

The Consumers' Association publishes the monthly journal *Which?* and also produces the *Drug and Therapeutics Bulletin* for the medical and allied professions. This Bulletin reports mainly on drugs, occasionally on minor items of medical equipment, appraises manufacturers' claims and compares new treatments with established ones used for the same conditions.

The Council for Music in Hospitals

6 Raymond Buildings, Gray's Inn, London, WC1.

The objects of the Council for Music in Hospitals are to encourage, counsel and assist the recovery of all persons, whether mentally or physically unwell, by the use of live concerts of good music as a therapeutic agent. Artists, including the famous, give their services for considerably reduced fees. Hospitals can be assisted in organizing lectures, meetings of gramophone clubs and similar activities on request.

The Crediton Project

West Longsight, Crediton, Devon.

The Crediton Project, a registered charity, promotes, in suitable cases, voluntary male sterilization by vasectomy as a method of birth control in the United Kingdom. It provides information and advice to persons interested in this subject.

Cystic Fibrosis Research Trust

5 Blyth Road, Bromley, Kent, BR1 3RS Tel no: 01 464 7211.

The Cystic Fibrosis Research Trust was founded in 1964 to finance research to find a complete cure and, in the meantime, to improve upon current methods of treatment; to establish branches and groups throughout the United Kingdom for the purpose of helping and advising parents with the everyday problems of caring for children with cystic fibrosis; to educate the public about the disease and, through increased knowledge, help to promote earlier diagnosis in young children.

Disabled Drivers' Association
Ashwellthorpe Road, Norwich, NR16 1EX
Tel no: 0508 41449.

The Disabled Drivers' Association exists to protect the interests of the physically handicapped on all matters connected with mobility, providing personal advice and guidance. It has sixty-six branches offering a variety of social activities, and on a national basis regular contacts are maintained with government departments, manufacturers and local authorities.

Disabled Living Foundation
346, Kensington High Street, London, W14 8NS
Tel no: 01 602 2491.

The Disabled Living Foundation is a registered charity which is concerned with the investigation of the problems of disabled people in the widest sense. Present projects include studies on the design of equipment, clothing problems, incontinence, gardening, physical recreation and music.

An Information Service for the Disabled is run on a subscription basis. Further details about subscription rates can be obtained from the DLF.

A comprehensive standing exhibition of aids of all kinds can be seen and demonstrated, preferably by prior appointment if possible.

Disablement Income Group – DIG
Queen's House, 180–182, Tottenham Court Road, London,
W1P 0BD Tel no: 01 636 1946/7.

The Disablement Income Group, DIG, is an action group formed to bring pressure to bear on the Government into implementing its policies for economic justice for all physically and mentally handicapped people in Great Britain.

Its aims are:

To secure the provision for all disabled people of a national disability income and an allowance for the extra expense of disablement.

To co-operate with other bodies working in the field for the improvement of the economic and social position of disabled people and the chronic sick.

To promote research into the economic and social problems of disablement.

It publishes a quarterly journal, *Progress*, and runs an advisory service. There are over fifty branches in the United Kingdom.

DIG's Charitable Trust is registered under the Charities Act 1960, No 251999. It has published *An ABC of Services and General Information for Disabled People*.

The Employment Fellowship
Drayton House, Gordon Street, London, WC1H 0BE
Tel no: 01 387 1828.

The Employment Fellowship has as its object to utilize the willingness of the elderly who wish to be employed on tasks adjusted to their strength and skill. It has applied its experience and resources in developing sheltered work centres which offer them companionship, useful occupation and supplementary income.

Family Planning Association
Margaret Pyke House, 27–35 Mortimer Street, London, W1A 4QW Tel no: 01 636 7866.

The Family Planning Association exists to help people have children only when they want them. It is a voluntary organization and a registered charity, with a record of 50 years' service to the public. It is one of the largest medical agencies in this country outside the National Health Service and over the years has built up a nation-wide professional clinic service for people with a wide range of needs.

The Haemophilia Society
16 Trinity Street, London, SE1 1DE Tel no: 01 407 1010.

The Haemophilia Society is a nationwide organization to provide fellowship for haemophiliacs, their families, friends and those interested in their health and welfare. The Society seeks to safeguard the social and economic interests of haemophiliacs and to promote the study of the causes and treatment of haemophilia and allied conditions. It offers practical help and advice on all problems likely to be encountered by a haemophiliac.

Handicapped Adventure Playground Association
203 King's Road, London, SW3. Tel no: 01 352 2321.

The object of the Handicapped Adventure Playground Association is to make provision, through the medium of play, for children and young people with mental, physical or emotional handicaps including those of vision, hearing and perception; to evolve, establish, develop and maintain adventure playgrounds especially designed to give enjoyment as well as sensory-motor training to the handicapped; to foster the interest of the public in the problems of the handicapped and to establish good contact with medical, teaching and research bodies, co-operating fully with them in the management and development of adventure playgrounds for the handicapped; to enable interested persons to gain first-hand experience of the emotional and therapeutic advantages obtainable through creative play.

The Hospital Saving Association
30 Lancaster Gate, London, W2 3LT Tel no: 01 723 7601.

The Hospital Saving Association is the largest hospital contributory scheme in the United Kingdom, with almost a million members. Their contributions ensure hospital, dental, optical and other benefits for the whole family. Founded in 1922, it is a non-profit-making body still financially supporting hospitals by annual grants to their free funds and through its awards of HSA scholarships for state registered nurses.

Ileostomy Association of Great Britain and Ireland
Drove Cottage, Fuzzy Drove, Kempshott, Basingstoke
Tel no: Basingstoke 21288.

The Ileostomy Association was formed to help ileostomists enjoy a full life and to deal with problems of employment, rehabilitation and social questions. It also promotes and co-ordinates research, collates records and improves knowledge of ileostomy techniques and appliances. A quarterly journal, containing articles of practical value and an exchange of views and experiences, is issued to members. The Kingston Trust (q.v.) runs special homes for ileostomists, providing convalescent and holiday accommodation as well as permanent homes for elderly ileostomists.

The Industrial Society
Robert Hyde House, 48 Bryanston Square, London, W1H 8AH Tel no: 01 262 2401.

The Industrial Society is an independent body founded to promote fuller involvement of people in their work as a means of increasing their personal satisfaction and the efficiency of the organization. Its services include courses and conferences; training within companies; advisory visits, information, publications, film-strips and a monthly magazine. It specializes in effective leadership, relations between management and unions, communication and involvement, conditions of employment, and the development of young employees. Members include industrial and commercial companies, central and local government departments, nationalized industries, trade unions and employers' associations. The Society's Public Services group provides a wide range of training and advisory services for hospitals and the health departments of local authorities on all aspects of the management of staff. Information on these subjects is available to member organizations from the Society's Information Department.

Institute for the Study of Drug Dependence
Kingsbury House, 3 Blackburn Road, London, NW6 1XA Tel no: 01 328 5541/2.

The Institute for the Study of Drug Dependence, founded in 1968, is an independent body whose main functions are to provide objective information, promote research in the field of drug dependence, and advance public understanding of the subject. A comprehensive information service is maintained. Requests for information are welcome, but should be as specific as possible. Reading lists will be supplied to those

wanting general background information. The Institute does
not treat addicts, nor does it give medical or legal advice.
It is, however, able to provide information on the facilities
and resources available.

Invalids-at-Home
23 Farm Avenue, London, NW2 2BJ. Tel no: 01 452 2074.
This organization aims to help permanent invalids, no
matter what the nature of their illness or disablement, to
leave hospital for home and to remain at home in greater
comfort and security.

It makes grants and interest-free loans, and many of the
larger amounts involved are to help disabled people continue
to earn their living – e.g. repair spares to help a man restart
his business, a high quality tape recorder to enable a broad-
caster and journalist to record at home, a car hoist without
which another man could not have used his car and travelled
to his place of business, and adaptations about the house to
assist a disabled housewife.

International Planned Parenthood Federation
18–20 Lower Regent Street, London, SW1 4PW
Tel no: 01 839 2911.
The International Planned Parenthood Federation is an
international non-governmental organization which encourages the formation of national family planning associations to pioneer family planning services and to bring about a
favourable climate of public opinion.

Family Planning Associations offer contraceptive services,
train all levels of personnel, and carry out education programmes to inform and teach people about the personal,
health, social and economic benefits of family planning and
responsible parenthood. The IPPF stimulates appropriate
scientific research in the following subjects: the biological,
demographic, social, economic, eugenic and psychological
implications of human fertility and its regulation; methods
of contraception; fertility, sub-fertility and sterility; sex
education, and marriage counselling. It collects and makes
known the findings of such research.

International Voluntary Service
91 High Street, Harlesden, London, NW10
Tel no: 01 965 1446.
International Voluntary Service is the British branch of Service Civil International, a worldwide organization with more than fifty years' experience of work to render war and the degradation of human dignity impossible through practical service to the community. IVS serves the community through the integrated action of its seventy-five local groups, international work camps at home and abroad, and through long term volunteers in Africa and Asia. Its members play with children, help the elderly and handicapped through gardening and decorating and work with hospitals, in the belief that it is possible for individuals to work together for peace, through a deepened understanding of society and an acceptance of a common humanity.

Invalid Children's Aid Association
126 Buckingham Palace Road, London, SW1W 9SB
Tel no: 01 730 9891.
The Invalid Children's Aid Association provides support and help of all kinds for families with a chronic sick or handicapped child. This is given through counselling by trained social workers, a postal information service, special schools and centres for handicaps not otherwise catered for, and financial help in special cases. Research and the training of students are an important part of the Association's work, and close contact is maintained with other welfare services.

Kids
17 Sedlescombe Road, London, SW6 1RE
Tel no: 01 381 0335.
Kids, a national society for deprived and handicapped children, recently completed a purpose-built Holiday Centre for deprived and handicapped children at Easton Maudit, Wellingborough, Northamptonshire. The Holiday Centre is open throughout the year, has a fully qualified staff and accommodates twelve children. The Centre will provide holidays for socially and physically handicapped children. Further details are obtainable from the Director.

The Kingston Trust
The Drove, Kempshott, Basingstoke, Hants
Tel no: Basingstoke 21288.

The Kingston Trust, founded in 1962, provides permanent and convalescent homes for 'stoma cases' with ileostomies, ileal bladders and colostomies. In affiliation with the Ileostomy Association (q.v.), the Trust also gives assistance in welfare and care to those patients in later life who are in need of help, priority being given to the elderly with ileostomies.

The Wallace-Kingston Trust was founded in 1972, to provide further help both in the homes of the Kingston Trust and for welfare generally to younger patients with abdominal diseases in need of care and understanding.

The Lady Hoare Trust for Thalidomide and Other Physically Disabled Children
7 North Street, Midhurst, Sussex. Tel no: Midhurst 4235.

The Lady Hoare Trust has been in existence since 1962 when Lady Hoare launched a national appeal for children damaged by the drug thalidomide. Since then, families have been sustained by the Trust, both financially and through a unique system of rehabilitation whereby they are helped and guided by Lady Hoare's team of twenty-six professional welfare visitors.

The Trust has introduced many revolutionary ideas, such as powered limbs and specially designed mini-cars which children, however badly disabled, can drive. The Trust also has many new projects, including four holiday homes, and advanced scientific educational aids which enable disabled children to keep up with normal children at school.

The Society for the Aid of Thalidomide Children, of which Lady Hoare was the Chairman before her death, is the parents' Society.

London Council of Social Service
68 Charlton Street, London, NW1 1JR Tel no: 01 388 0241.

The London Council of Social Service supports voluntary social and community work agencies, encouraging coordination and co-operation with statutory agencies. It has specialist staff working in the following fields: community

330

A Guide to other available help

development, training, race relations, work with homeless families, and development of opportunities for voluntary work. The Council supports councils of social service in many London boroughs, and provides the secretariat for the Greater London Standing Conference of Voluntary Youth Organizations.

Marie Curie Memorial Foundation
124 Sloane Street, London, SW1X 9BP Tel no: 01 730 9157.
The Marie Curie Memorial Foundation, working solely in the cancer field, provides throughout the United Kingdom (a) 414 beds for seriously ill or convalescent cancer patients distributed in twelve nursing homes; (b) a professional day and night nursing service for patients in their own homes; and (c) a welfare grant scheme providing urgent necessities in kind. It maintains a central advisory and education bureau, and has established a rehabilitation centre attached to one of its homes. Research into human cancer is undertaken at its own research laboratories.

Medic-Alert Foundation
9 Hanover Street, London, W1R 9HF Tel no: 01 499 2261.
The Medic-Alert Foundation provides any person with a hidden medical problem with the protection of an emblem which gives an immediate warning to hospitals, doctors, police, or others who might attend them at a time when they are unable to speak for themselves, e.g. an accident. The Foundation provides a bracelet or necklet with medical insignia on one side and the appropriate medical warning engraved on the reverse, and a serial number. A central file is maintained in London. In an emergency, information can be obtained by a doctor or other authorized person by making a reverse-charge telephone call from anywhere in the world. This service is 24-hours a day.

Medical Council on Alcoholism
8 Bourdon Street, Davies Street, London, W1 9HY
Tel no: 01 493 0081.
The Medical Council on Alcoholism has as its main aims education, research, and the production of information on all matters to do with alcoholism. It is anxious to obtain

recognition amongst the general public, industry, the Government and even doctors themselves, that alcoholism is a disease and, as such, both a clinical and community health problem. The Council produces a quarterly journal on alcoholism. A library and information service is available.

Medical Recording Service Foundation:
Royal College of General Practitioners
Kitts Croft, Writtle, Chelmsford, CM1 3EH.

The Medical Recording Service Foundation of the Royal College of General Practitioners provides a postal library, available at moderate charge to any medical worker. It comprises audiovisual educational material – mainly audio tapes with accompanying slides. A wide range of subjects suitable for use by hospital doctors, nurses and for educating school children, is covered. Sets of slides, for use by teachers to illustrate their own teaching, are available. A library list which describes individual talks and the audiences for whom they are designed is also available.

Medical Research Council
20 Park Crescent, London, W1N 4AL Tel no: 01 636 5422.

The Medical Research Council is the main government agency for the promotion of medical research. It is financed by an annual grant-in-aid from Parliament. The Council's constitution gives it full liberty to pursue an independent policy for the advancement of knowledge towards the relief of human suffering, and its particular role is to assist the balanced development of medical and related biological research in the country as a whole by providing support complementary to the resources of the universities and hospitals. The Council employs its own research staff; it also awards long-term and project research grants and offers fellowships and scholarships for training in research.

The Mental After Care Association
Eagle House, 110 Jermyn Street, London, SW1Y 6HB Tel no: 01 839 5953.

The Mental After Care Association provides rehabilitation hostels for mentally convalescent men and women of working age and capacity who need a sympathetic home environment and skilled help in getting suitable employment and making satisfactory social adjustments; long-stay homes for elderly, mentally-disturbed people who do not need to remain in hospital but require skilled supervision and trained care to enable them to live as independently as their condition allows; holiday accommodation for psychiatric hospital patients not yet fit for discharge but able to enjoy a 'break'; and for those whose relatives need some respite from the burden of caring for them at home.

The Migraine Trust
23 Queen Square, London, WC1N 3AY Tel no: 01 278 2676.

The Migraine Trust, a registered charity, was founded in 1965 to finance and co-ordinate research into the causes, treatment and cure of migraine. It also provides sufferers with information and advice. International symposia are held for those engaged in research into migraine.

The largest and most ambitious of the Trust's current research projects is the City Migraine Clinic, 11–12, Bartholomew Close, London, EC1 (Tel no: 01 606 1643) which primarily exists for examining and treating patients in an attack. It also sees patients, free of charge, following a letter from their doctor. *Hemicrania* is published quarterly for the medical profession. *Migraine News* is issued to subscribers.

The Multiple Sclerosis Society
4 Tachbrook Street, London, SW1V 1SJ
Tel no: 01 834 8231/2/3.

The Multiple Sclerosis Society has as its aims the encouragement of research into the causes and cure of multiple sclerosis, and helps persons suffering from the disease, co-operating with welfare authorities through countrywide branches. In co-operation with local authorities, the Society is making purpose-built accommodation available near to established and planned day care centres. These projects have been specially designed to aid patients and their families so that partners continue in employment and the patient is well catered for during the day in the nearby day care centre.

Muscular Dystrophy Group of Great Britain
26 Borough High Street, London, SE1 9QG
Tel no: 01 407 5116.

The Muscular Dystrophy Group of Great Britain exists to finance research into the cure and treatment of muscular dystrophy and allied diseases. Branches throughout the country provide a friendly link between sufferers, as well as organizing fund-raising activities. Welfare work is also carried out within the branches and the Group administers a small welfare fund. Welfare matters may be referred to the Group's Medical Social Worker.

National Addiction and Research Institute
533a King's Road, London, SW10 Tel no: 01 352 1590 and 4517.

CURE, the National Addiction and Research Institute, is a centre drawing on various professions for the treatment of those addicted to drugs. It specializes in the treatment of those using more than one drug, before they have reached the stage where they need care at a government centre, or on rehabilitation, when, after being in hospital or prison, they become free of drugs.

The rehabilitation centre, the Here and Now, led by a group of ex-addicts, is a place where those who have stopped using drugs can learn to become useful members of society by working in a therapeutic community. Members are expected to participate in a reassessment of their style of life. They can take part in activities including art and drama therapy, film making, screen printing and pottery. Special emphasis is placed on family therapy, and other forms of treatment, where the participation of selected groups in their own treatment is undertaken. The Institute undertakes educational work, such as training visits for people with professional interests, and is involved in a number of courses in conjunction with the Polytechnic of Central London concerning the abuse of drugs.

National Association for Maternity and Child Welfare
Tavistock House North, Tavistock Square, London,
WC1H 9JG Tel no: 01 387 1874.

The primary object of the National Association for Maternity and Child Welfare is to further education in this field.

Conferences are held annually in London and other cities. The majority of local health authorities in Great Britain are affiliated to it, and membership is open to teaching hospital groups, hospital management committees and individual maternity and child welfare centres. Overseas contacts are maintained. The Association suggests syllabuses for use in schools, colleges and clubs. It runs an advisory service and parentcraft classes for boys and girls. Examinations are held and graded certificates of instruction are awarded to successful candidates.

The Association also publishes a wide range of booklets and leaflets on maternity and child welfare. A publications list may be obtained from the above address.

National Association for the Welfare of Children in Hospital
Exton House, 7 Exton Street, London, SE1 8VE
Tel no: 01 261 1738.

The National Association for the Welfare of Children in Hospital was founded in 1961 to persuade hospitals that parents have a role to play in the care of children in hospital, and to persuade parents to take up that role. NAWCH promotes the need for fully unrestricted visiting, living-in accommodation for mothers, provision for play, suitable accident/emergency and out-patient facilities, an extension of home care services, and a considerable improvement in the quality of life for children in long stay wards. The Association organizes hospital play schemes and transport services, provides furnishings and equipment for wards and mothers' units, surveys facilities for visiting and play, maintains an information service and publishes leaflets, comics and painting books to help prepare children for hospital. It arranges conferences and promotes research on topics of current interest.

Similar organizations have been set up in Australia, Canada, Denmark, Eire, New Zealand, Norway, Sweden and the USA.

National Association of Leagues of Hospital Friends
44 Fulham Road, London, SW3 6HH Tel no: 01 584 7713.

The objects of the National Association of Leagues of Hospital Friends are threefold; to encourage, foster and maintain the interest of the public in the patients and staff of their local hospitals; to provide amenities and extra comforts for patients and staff, and to supplement the resources of the hospital service; and to recruit, and assist in the recruitment of, voluntary workers in, and for, local hospitals.

National Association of Voluntary Help Organizers
c/o The Voluntary Service Information Officer, The King's Fund Centre, 24 Nutford Place, London, W1H 6AN Tel no: 01 262 2641.
The Standing Conference of Voluntary Help Organizers was established in 1968. At the Annual General Meeting of this Conference on 15 February 1973 it was renamed the National Association of Voluntary Help Organizers. Its main purpose is to assist with the setting up of effective voluntary help schemes in hospitals, social services departments and the community. Full membership, which is by election, is open to formally appointed Voluntary Help Organizers or Co-ordinators. Associate membership is offered to people working with volunteers but who do not qualify for full membership. Information leaflets on Policy, Guidelines, New Appointments, Training and Salaries are available from the Hon. Secretary.

The National Childbirth Trust
9 Queensborough Terrace, London, W2 3TB Tel no: 01 229 9319/9310.
The National Childbirth Trust is a voluntary organization which promotes preparation for parenthood through classes at its headquarters and in its many branches. It publishes books and pamphlets for ante-natal teachers and parents, and offers seminar courses, study days and conferences for teachers, and film shows for teachers, parents-to-be, and young people.

National Children's Bureau
8 Wakley Street, London, EC1V 7QE Tel no: 01 278 9441.
The National Children's Bureau is an inter-professional organization concerned with children. Its activities include

336

research, such as the National Child Development Study; publications, like the research reviews on *The Handicapped Child, Living with Handicap,* and *The Challenge of Thalidomide,* and books in the series *Studies in Child Development*; an information service for professional workers about new developments or modifications of services for children, references, documentary films, and production of the *Spotlight* series of information handbooks; setting up the Children's Centre; and annual conferences, regional groups, etc. Membership includes most local authorities, professional and voluntary organizations, University and College departments, consultative members including government departments, and individual members.

National Citizens' Advice Bureaux Council
26 Bedford Square, London, WC1B 3HU Tel no: 01 636 4066.

The National Citizens' Advice Bureaux Council is an independent, non-political organization with 570 offices all over the country. Its purpose is to make available to the individual accurate information and skilled advice on many of the personal problems that arise in daily life; to explain legislation; to help the citizen benefit from, and use wisely, the services provided for him by the State, and in general to provide counsel to men and women in the many difficulties which beset them. Free information and advice are given in confidence to any person on any question that they might wish to ask. This includes help with problems connected with house purchase, property and land, social insurance and benefits, how to obtain legal aid, consumer problems, hire purchase, family and personal problems, problems of marriage, difficulties with landlord, tenant or neighbour, eviction orders, family budgeting, employment, education and training, taxes and duties, insurance, health and medical matters.

The Council publishes leaflets on various practical problems, eg, *Buying a House or a Flat, The Divorce Reform Act, Practical Problems following a Death*; these are available at a small charge from local offices.

The National Council for Special Education
Beaconwood, Bordon Hill, Stratford-Upon-Avon, Warwicks Tel no: 021 7444 162.

The National Council for Special Education exists to further the education and welfare of handicapped children, whatever the severity or type of disability. It consists mainly of teachers engaged in special education, but includes also some medical officers, psychologists, social workers, therapists and administrators. There are 50 branches covering most parts of Great Britain. The Council publishes a quarterly journal, *Special Education*, and a newsletter.

The National Council for the Single Woman and her Dependants
166 Victoria Street, London, SW1 Tel no: 01 828 5511.

The National Council for the Single Woman and Her Dependants provides an advisory centre for single women who have undertaken the care of infirm or elderly dependants. The Council seeks to ensure that welfare services are fitted to their needs. It has a small fund from which it provides interest-free loans to help meet financial crises, and seeks further social security benefits for single women caring for the aged infirm at home. The Council hopes to set up housing, with wardens on call, for single women going out to work and leaving an elderly dependant at home. It is also concerned with the problems of single women after the death of their dependants. There are branches throughout the UK. A bi-monthly newsletter is distributed.

National Council for Voluntary Youth Services
26 Bedford Square, London, WC1B 3HU Tel no: 01 636 4066.

The National Council for Voluntary Youth Services (formerly the Standing Conference of National Voluntary Youth Organizations) is a co-ordinating body, comprising the major voluntary youth organizations in the country. The present membership is fifty-nine youth organizations or agencies, and nine observers. The Council exists to strengthen and support the work of its members in endeavouring to meet the needs and aspirations of young people. It publishes a quarterly journal, and issues an annual directory free of charge.

National Deaf Children's Society
31 Gloucester Place, London, W1H 4EA
Tel no: 01 486 3251/2.

The National Deaf Children's Society exists to promote the maximum benefit and happiness for all deaf children through their home environment, their education, and the co-operation of the general public. On the advice of medical and educational research committees, the Society promotes and finances medical and educational research in all aspects of the handicap. There are fifty-five regional associations in England, Scotland, Wales and Northern Ireland.

National Elfrida Rathbone Society
17 Victoria Park Square, London, E2 Tel no: 01 980 4204.

The National Elfrida Rathbone Society is a central voluntary organization concerned with the provision of social facilities for educationally subnormal children and their families. The Society works through local groups to promote action within the community, relying largely, though not entirely, on the help and skill of volunteers. Each local group is independent, carrying out whatever projects are within its capabilities and appropriate to its particular area. Examples of such projects include youth clubs, holiday schemes, literacy projects, voluntary home visiting, pre-school playgroups and mothers' clubs. The Development Officers of the Society are responsible for supporting existing groups, and for initiating new work in areas where none exists at present.

National Federation of Clubs for the Divorced and Separated
13 High Street, Little Shelford, Cambridge
Tel no: Shelford 2544.

The aims of the National Federation of Clubs for the Divorced and Separated are to promote the proper interests of divorced and separated people and to provide a channel for the formation and representation of opinion on matters of common concern; to provide a central register of *bona fide* clubs for the information of divorced and separated people and for social workers in official and voluntary agencies. The Clubs provide a social outlet, and it is hoped that through their agency the genuine needs of divorced and

339

separated people may be recognized more clearly. There is no discrimination of sex, race, politics or religion.

National Federation of Women's Institutes
39 Eccleston Street, Victoria, London, SW1W 9NT
Tel no: 01 730 7212.

The original object of the National Federation of Women's Institutes was 'to improve and develop conditions of rural life', though the work now encompasses many aspects of working nationally and internationally, and there are now Women's Institutes in many towns and cities. It provides for the education of women in citizenship, practical skills and cultural subjects. There are now thirty-seven Institutes in psychiatric hospitals, eleven in hospitals for the mentally sub-normal, one in a hostel for the mentally sub-normal, one in a hostel for disabled girls, one in a hostel for epileptics, one in a geriatric hospital and two in Cheshire Homes. Others help by befriending and entertaining patients in similar hospitals.

National Innovations Centre
Bedford Chambers, Covent Garden, London, WC2E 8HA
Tel no: 01 836 8967.

The function of the National Innovations Centre (NIC), formerly the National Suggestions Centre, is to seek out schemes which break new ground in the field of social welfare, to spread information about them, and to promote their wider adoption, either by voluntary or by statutory bodies. Emphasis is given to projects which make a special contribution to the welfare of selected groups, notably the aged, the sick and the isolated.

The National Marriage Guidance Council
Herbert Gray College, Little Church Street, Rugby,
Warwickshire Tel no: Rugby 73241.

The National Marriage Guidance Council offers four main services: private counselling for people who have difficulties or anxieties in their marriage or in other personal relationships; discussion with small groups of young people or with engaged and young married couples; publication of non-technical, but authoritative and practical, booklets on a wide variety of topics connected with marriage and family life; courses and conferences for teachers, clergy, youth leaders and others.

National Research Development Corporation
Kingsgate House, 66–74 Victoria Street, London, SW1E 6SL Tel no: 01 828 3400.

The National Research Development Corporation is a public corporation which provides financial and other support for technological developments of potential commercial importance, and promotes the adoption by industry of new products and processes invented in government laboratories, universities, medical schools, hospitals, and other health establishments.

The National Society for Autistic Children
1a Golders Green Road, London, NW11 Tel no: 01 458 4375.

The National Society for Autistic Children seeks to provide and promote day and residential centres for the care and education of autistic children. It helps parents by arranging meetings where they can exchange information with other parents, encourages research into the problems of these children, and endeavours to stimulate greater understanding of their difficulties amongst doctors, teachers and the general public. There is an advisory service for parents, and an information service for professional people. The Society publishes and distributes literature on the management and education of autistic children.

National Society for Cancer Relief
Michael Sobell House, 30 Dorset Square, London, NW1 6QL Tel no: 01 402 8125.

The National Society for Cancer Relief has as its object the relief of distress, anxiety and fear among cancer patients and their families. It makes grants to enable patients to buy extra food, fuel, clothing, special equipment and other necessities, to pay nursing-home fees and to assist with fares for those visiting patients in hospital. It pays expenses in whole, or in part, for convalescent holidays and it helps to provide necessary attention such as domestic help and skilled home nursing for those discharged from hospital. It also makes substantial contributions to the building costs of nursing homes for cancer sufferers.

National Society for Clean Air
136 North Street, Brighton, Sussex, BN1 1RG
Tel no: Brighton 26313/4/5.

The aims of the National Society for Clean Air are to promote and create by publicity and education an informed public opinion on the value and importance of clean air, and to initiate, promote and encourage the investigation and research into all forms of atmospheric pollution in order to achieve its reduction or prevention. The Society's main activities are the holding of conferences, meetings and exhibitions; arranging lectures; providing educational and publicity material and collecting and disseminating information in the form of books, pamphlets, periodicals, photographs and slides about the causes, effects and prevention of atmospheric pollution. The annual conference proceedings are published as well as the *Clean Air Year Book* and a quarterly journal, *Clean Air*.

National Society for Mentally Handicapped Children
5 Coventry Street, London, W1 Tel no: 01 437 4538.

The National Society for Mentally Handicapped Children is a voluntary organization of parents with 35,000 members in 400 Local Societies. Twelve regional officers support their activities and undertake liaison with statutory authorities. The Society organizes welfare, research, residential centres, speech therapy, physiotherapy, a trusteeship scheme, youth clubs, a bookshop, courses and seminars.

National Society for the Prevention of Cruelty to Children
1 Riding House Street, London, W1P 8AA
Tel no: 01 580 8812.

The National Society for the Prevention of Cruelty to Children exists to help any child in this country whatever his colour, nationality or creed and any parent with a problem concerning the welfare of their children or their family. The Society works with families in their own homes, striving always to keep the family together; it investigates reports of neglect or ill-treatment of children.

National Society of Non-Smokers
125 West Dumpton Lane, Ramsgate
Tel no: Thanet 55036.
The National Society of Non-Smokers, upholding the interests of non-smokers, questions the right of smokers to pollute the communal atmosphere in enclosed public places, including hospitals. It has secured the restriction of smoking in trains, buses, airliners, theatres and hotels.

Nuffield Nursing Homes Trust
10 Essex Street, London, WC2R 3AX Tel no: 01 353 9451.
Founded in 1957 by the British United Provident Association Limited (BUPA), the Nuffield Nursing Homes Trust now has twenty homes in operation throughout the country, providing over 600 up-to-date private beds for more than 21,000 in-patients a year. Six more Trust homes are now in various stages of development. The Trust's long-term goal is the establishment, within the bounds of available finance, of nursing homes for surgical and medical patients.

Nursery School Association of Great Britain and Northern Ireland
89 Stamford Street, London, SE1 Tel no: 01 928 7454.
The Nursery School Association of Great Britain and Northern Ireland offers advice on nursery and infant education and on the training of teachers and nursery assistants. It encourages local authorities to provide for nursery education and makes its contribution in the field of nursery and infant education by means of conferences, schools and publications. A summer school is held each year and an international one in alternate years. Its various committees include those on finance, publications, courses and conferences, private nurseries and research. There is also a medical committee and a buildings advisory committee.

Nursing and Hospital Careers Information Centre
121–123 Edgware Road, London, W2 Tel no: 01 402 5296/7.
The Nursing and Hospital Careers Information Centre is a centre where people can call between the hours of 10 am and 5 pm, Monday to Friday, without making an appointment, to discuss nursing and other hospital careers with an Information Officer. Enquiries can also be made by telephone or letter. The Centre provides a place where those engaged in careers advisory work and recruitment can meet to discuss their plans and obtain up-to-date information.

The Optical Information Council
Aldwych House, Aldwych, London, WC2 B4HN
Tel no: 01 242 5146/7.
The Optical Information Council is supported by voluntary subscribers from the optical profession and industry. It was formed in 1951 as a non-profit-making body, and provides information on all matters relating to the function and care of sight and the products of the ophthalmic industry.

Paintings in Hospitals
Nuffield Foundation, Nuffield Lodge, Regent's Park, London, NW1 4RS Tel no: 01 722 8871.
Paintings in Hospitals is an organization which lends modern original paintings and lithographs to hospitals in the London area. The scheme is expanding to include other parts of the country, and pilot schemes are being started in Cambridge and Glasgow. A fee of £1.00 per annum for each picture is charged to cover insurance, transport and repair costs.

Parkinson's Disease Society of the United Kingdom Limited
81 Queens Road, Wimbledon, London, SW19 8NR
Tel no: 01 946 2500.
Parkinson's Disease Society is a registered charity. Its principal objects are: (a) to help patients and their families with problems arising from the disease; (b) to collect and publish information about it; and (c) to sponsor research from monies raised.

The Patients Association
335 Grays Inn Road, London, WC1X 8PX
Tel no: 01 837 7241.
The Patients Association represents and furthers the interests of patients generally, and assists and advises individual patients. Constant contact with patients enables it to advise hospital authorities on patients' views, problems and reactions. The Association also provides speakers to address nurses, administrators and other interested people.

Photography for the Disabled
190 Secrett House, Ham Close, Ham, Richmond, Surrey
Tel no: 01 948 2342.
Photography for the Disabled has as its purpose to promote the welfare of handicapped persons by providing cameras and other photographic equipment suitably adapted to meet their individual needs and so enable them to practise photography.

Possum Users Association
'Kerridge', 25 World's End Lane, Weston Turville, Aylesbury, Bucks, HP22 5SA Tel no: 612235.
The aim of the Possum Users Association is to assist people who are severely physically disabled in gaining independence, and thus the possibility of communication, education and employment. The Association provides information and advice by newsletter for the benefit of its members. It raises funds to supply special equipment for the disabled, and co-operates with other associations in improving social and economic conditions. The Association is run in an entirely honorary capacity by severely disabled people who themselves use Possum equipment.

Pre-School Playgroups Association
Alford House, Aveline Street, London, SE11 5DJ
Tel no: 01 582 8871.
The Pre-school Playgroups Association promotes the formation of playgroups for children primarily from three to five years old, and encourages the study of the needs and problems of all pre-school children. Among the needs of

345

children in hospital is that of play, and the Association encourages the provision of good play facilities and skilled supervision for these children.

Psychiatric Rehabilitation Association
21a, Kingsland High Street, Dalston, London, E8
Tel no: 01 254 9753 and 01 249 0957.

The purpose of the Psychiatric Rehabilitation Association is to stimulate the patient towards greater initiative and social awareness of his environment and society. It encourages and prepares him to return and readapt to his community. At the same time, the Association seeks to improve attitudes towards the mentally ill and promotes practical measures for preventing and combating mental distress within the community. Its wide range of services include research projects, training programmes for volunteers, holiday schemes, home visiting, industrial education units, day centres, a Sunday lunch club, a residential centre, and group homes.

Release
1 Elgin Avenue, London, W9 Tel no: 01 289 1123 Emer.
Tel no: 01 603 8654.

Release gives advice to young people on legal and medical problems including arrest on drug or other charges, adverse drug reactions, psychiatric problems, pregnancy and accommodation. Factual information on abuse of drugs and related topics is also given. Referral to solicitors, doctors, psychiatrists, and other professional help, is available any time during office hours which are from 10.00 am–6.00 pm Monday to Friday and until 10.00 pm on Mondays and Thursdays. An emergency service by telephone (no: 01 603 8654) is run 24-hours a day.

Responaut
39 Essex Street, Newbury, Berkshire.

The Responaut is a journal published quarterly for the purposes of restoring natural liberties to disabled people by showing the strengths and weaknesses of welfare services, statutory, voluntary and commercial, and to discuss equipment and ideas to fill the gaps. *The Responaut* is able to maintain its completely independent position because all articles and photographs are contributed free and the publication is printed and posted without charge by IPC on the grounds that 'the biggest and strongest must help the smallest and weakest'. Government ministers, Members of Parliament, engineers, hospital specialists and therapists, domiciliary workers and disabled people contribute to, and read, *The Responaut.*

Riding for the Disabled Association
National Equestrian Centre, Kenilworth, Warwickshire, CV8 2LR Tel no: Coventry 27192.

The Riding for the Disabled Association has for its purpose to provide facilities for riding for all disabled people who may wish to do so and have been given medical approval. It has been shown over the past twenty years that even severely handicapped people can gain much pleasure and satisfaction from learning to ride, and many acquire considerable skill in spite of the difficulties. The mobility and freedom provided by a pony are particularly valuable to children whose normal range of movement is restricted to a wheelchair or crutches. The Association is a registered charity with about 180 component groups in the United Kingdom.

Royal Association in Aid of the Deaf and Dumb
7 Armstrong Road, Acton, London, W3 7JL Tel no: 01 743 6187/8.

The Royal Association in Aid of the Deaf and Dumb works in London, Essex, Surrey and West Kent with the men and women who have been deaf since childhood and especially with those who cannot communicate adequately by speech. The Association also works with those who are deaf and blind, and with deaf patients in mental hospitals. Through its trained staff and its special churches and social clubs, the Association strives to help deaf people to help themselves achieve their full personal development and reach their highest potential as members of the community.

The Royal College of Nursing and National Council of Nurses of the United Kingdom
1, Henrietta Place, Cavendish Square, London, W1M 0AB Tel no: 01 580 2646.

The Royal College of Nursing is the professional organization for registered, enrolled, student, and pupil nurses, and now has over 100,000 members. It is concerned with promoting higher standards of nursing care, the better education and training of nurses, and the advancement of the profession. It is a certificate-granting body, and is recognized by the Department of Education and Science as a major establishment of further education for nurses. It negotiates salaries and conditions of service and provides free protection, representation, and advice on professional problems for all members. It keeps under review all matters which may affect the profession, and the service it gives to the community. It also provides a Welfare Advisory Service for all nurses, whether or not they are RCN members, who are in personal or financial difficulty.

The Royal National Institute for the Blind
224 Great Portland Street, London, W1N 6AA Tel no: 01 388 1266.

The Royal National Institute for the Blind looks after all aspects of welfare for the blind of all ages. It runs the Queen Elizabeth Homes of Recovery, Sunshine Homes, schools for blind babies and children, rehabilitation centres for the newly blind, and homes for the elderly blind. Braille and Moon books and periodicals, talking books, Braille music and apparatus and appliances for the blind and deaf-blind are provided. It sponsors scientific and mechanical research and gives professional and technical training for physiotherapy, commercial and industrial occupations.

Royal National Institute for the Deaf
105 Gower Street, London, WC1E 6AH Tel no: 01 387 8033.

The Royal National Institute for the Deaf, founded in 1911, is the protective association for all deaf and hard-of-hearing people in the United Kingdom. As well as representing their interests it gives advice and information on all matters concerning deafness and hearing. It operates six homes, mainly for the elderly, a training centre for maladjusted young deaf men, a hostel for working young deaf men, and a school for maladjusted deaf children. The services of its library are available to members of the public. The technical department advises on hearing aids, which it tests free of charge. The social work department augments the services of local authorities in London and gives help to those writing to the Institute about difficulties.

Royal Society for the Prevention of Accidents
Royal Oak Centre, Brighton Road, Purley, Surrey, CR2 2UR Tel no: 01 668 4272.

The Royal Society for the Prevention of Accidents is concerned with education for safety and preventing accidents, through training and publicity in relation to homes, water, roads, industry and agriculture. The work of the Society is co-ordinated by the various divisions at Head Office and is also carried out locally by the various regional offices and committees. The Society is non-profit-making and relies mainly on income from subscriptions of members, other contributions and sales of publications.

The St John Ambulance Association and Brigade
St John Ambulance, 1 Grosvenor Crescent, London, SW1X 7EF Tel no: 01 235 5231.

The objects of St John are to spread a knowledge of first aid, nursing and allied subjects among the general public, and in industry, and to provide a voluntary practical service for the community. It organizes classes and examinations, issues government-recognized certificates to successful candidates, arranges competitions, publishes text books and develops training aids. The voluntary service is provided by uniformed members who are on duty wherever crowds gather. They help in hospitals, homes and clinics, escort sick and injured people by land, sea and air, and assist the elderly or incapacitated in their homes. St John cadets are prepared for service in the adult units.

The Samaritans
39 Walbrook, London, EC4 Tel no: 01 626 2277.
The Samaritans exist to befriend the suicidal and despairing. They advertise emergency numbers for 137 branches in the United Kingdom so that immediate contact can be made at any time of day or night. The clients' problems are treated in the strictest confidence. The Samaritans are lay people from all walks of life. They do not seek to convert their clients to any faith or point of view, but offer the friendship of fellow humans beings, supplemented, if necessary, by counselling from professional people or treatment by a doctor.

Sesame
George Bell House, Bishop's Hall, 8, Ayres Street, London, SE1 1ES Tel no: 01 407 2159.
Sesame encourages the mentally and physically sick and handicapped, the blind, deaf and elderly to take an active part in drama and so help them enjoy a fuller life through music and movement, mime and simple acting. It works through hospital boards and national organizations. Travelling groups entertain and involve their audiences. Training courses by professionals are offered to teachers and therapists and are adapted to the needs of the individual hospitals with special tuition on application. Sesame only undertakes scientifically controlled research in co-operation with hospitals and other centres.

The Shaftesbury Society
112 Regency Street, London, SW1P 4AX Tel no: 01 834 2656.
The Shaftesbury Society has for over eighty years provided special residential care and teaching for disabled children. Although the Society provides for all types of physical disability there is a special responsibility for those suffering from either spina bifida or from muscular dystrophy. The Society now administers eight schools and homes where it seeks to provide higher standards of accommodation and personal care than can be found elsewhere. A new hostel has been built at Ossett in Yorkshire: it is for after-school care of the most severely handicapped.

Shelter, The National Campaign for the Homeless
86 Strand, London, WC2R 0EQ Tel no: 01 836 2051.
Shelter, The National Campaign for the Homeless, has rescued over 12,000 families since 1967; it campaigns intensively on behalf of the homeless, and supports experimental housing projects. SHAC, the Shelter Housing Aid Centre, 189a Old Brompton Road, London, SW5, provides comprehensive housing aid and advice for people living in London. It can advise on buying a house and obtaining a mortgage; help those wanting to move out of London; advise, and help, where possible, people needing to rent a flat in London. Membership is open to anyone wishing to join a Shelter Group or help in any other way.

Social Work Advisory Service
26 Bloomsbury Way, London, WC1A 2SR Tel no: 01 242 5654/5.
The Social Work Advisory Service is a centre for information on education, training and careers in the field of social work. The Service also has offices at Castlerock House, Castlerock, Co. Londonderry, N. Ireland, and 50, Queen Street, Edinburgh, EH2 3NS. Advice is given by letter, and interviews are arranged by appointment, at the three offices, and in a number of regional centres. Leaflets and booklets on various aspects of social work carried out by local authorities, the hospital service and voluntary organizations are available.

The Spastics Society
12 Park Crescent, London, W1N 4EQ Tel no: 01 636 5020.
In order to develop the potential of spastics, fifty per cent of whom suffer some degree of mental handicap, The Spastics Society has established skilled assessment and psychological services. The Society and its 176 affiliated local groups have built up a network of more than 140 schools, residential and day care centres, hostels, and training establishments for the welfare and education of spastics of all types and ages. The Society emphasizes social training to enable as many as possible to live within the community instead of in sub-normality hospitals.

Task Force
Clifford House, Edith Villas, W14 8UG.
Tel no: 01 602 2627.

Task Force has centres in ten London Boroughs: Barnet, Camden, Ealing, Greenwich, Hackney, Islington, Kensington and Chelsea, Lewisham, Wandsworth and Westminster. The centres are each manned by four full-time staff whose job it is to put young volunteers in touch with elderly people in need of friendship and practical help. The scheme began in October, 1964, and at present approximately 9,000 young people are helping 3,000 old people regularly in their own homes, hospitals and in homes. Task Force is also involved in teaching social education in schools, and researching into any needs it discovers.

Trans-Care International (Transport and Escort) Service
269–273 High Street, Croydon, CR0 1QH
Tel no: 01 686 0102.

Trans-Care International escorts and transports the sick, injured and disabled to and from anywhere in the United Kingdom, Europe, or the rest of the world. All categories of patients are dealt with and are transported by specially constructed long distance road ambulances and executive jet air ambulance. There is a 24-hour stand-by service with a multi-lingual staff. Nursing home facilities are available for overnight, short stay or accident treatment. Doctors and nurses are provided for escort by scheduled air or sea services.

The Voluntary Euthanasia Society
13 Prince of Wales Terrace, London, W8 5PG
Tel no: 01 937 7770.

The Voluntary Euthanasia Society has as its object to promote legislation which would give an adult, in carefully defined circumstances and with appropriate safeguards, the choice between prolonged suffering and gentle, dignified death. The Society's proposals are strictly voluntary for doctors, nurses and patients. No one would ever be called upon to act against his own conscience and principles. Literature is available free on request.

Women's Royal Voluntary Service
17 Old Park Lane, London, W1Y 4AJ Tel no: 01 499 6040.
Members of the Women's Royal Voluntary Service work in 1,496 hospitals in Great Britain including 121 psychiatric hospitals and 85 for the mentally handicapped. The aim is to add to the patients' welfare and relieve the staff of nonnursing duties. The work undertaken includes serving in canteens in outpatients' departments; static shops, trolley services to wards, shops and canteen units, and social clubs in psychiatric hospitals, and in hospitals for the mentally handicapped; reception and escorting of patients, and children's playgroups.

Special Schools for Handicapped Pupils
Local education authorities have a duty to provide special education for handicapped pupils. Ten categories of such pupils are defined in the Handicapped Pupils and Special Schools Regulations 1959 (as amended). These categories are: the physically handicapped, deaf, partially hearing, blind, partially sighted, educationally subnormal, epileptic, maladjusted, those suffering from speech defects not due to deafness, and the delicate. The Education (Handicapped Children) Act 1970, which came into force in April 1971, placed responsibility for the education of mentally handicapped children, as for children with any other handicap, with education authorities. Sections 25 to 27 of the Chronically Sick and Disabled Persons Act 1970 placed a duty on education authorities to provide special facilities for deaf blind and autistic children, and those suffering from dyslexia, as far as possible, in ordinary schools.

Seriously handicapped pupils are generally taught in special schools, either day or boarding. Special schools which are boarding are necessary for several reasons – e.g. the severity of the handicap; the small number of children suffering from certain handicaps, which makes local day school provision impracticable; and the existence of unsatisfactory home conditions. Most special day schools are, however, maintained by voluntary organizations. There are also special schools in hospitals where the number of long-term child patients makes it worthwhile.

Education is compulsory for children at special schools between the ages of five and sixteen. Normally, schooling does not begin before the age of five; but there are nursery schools for very young blind children who, for some reason, cannot be cared for at home and, with the increasing importance now attached to the early training and education of the deaf, most special schools for the deaf admit children from the age of two or three years.

There are one or two grammar schools for the blind and for the deaf to which selected children are admitted at the age of eleven or twelve years. These provide a mainly academic course, and pupils often remain until the age of eighteen or nineteen. There is also a selective school, providing secondary education up to the age of eighteen or nineteen for deaf boys, at which the courses have a technical or art bias.

Special educational treatment for the less seriously disabled may be provided in ordinary schools; maladjusted pupils, for example, may be given treatment by the child guidance staff of the local education authority and, if their home conditions demand it, live in special hostels or with foster parents.

In exceptional cases local education authorities may provide education other than at school, for example, at hospitals where there are too few patients to justify the establishment of a hospital special school or, where the circumstances justify it, in the child's home.

Addresses and Social Service Functions of Central Government Departments

Education and Science, Department of
Curzon Street, London, W1.
Educational services, including school meals and (until 1974) school medical services.
Scotland: *Scottish Education Department*, St Andrew's House, Edinburgh 1.
Wales: *Education Office for Wales*, 31 Cathedral Road, Cardiff.

Employment, Department of
8 St James Square, London, SW1.
Employment services, including employment exchanges and the special services for youth employment, disabled persons, industrial training, rehabilitation, safety, health and welfare at work.
Industrial relations between employer and employed.

Environment, Department of the
2 Marsham Street, London, SW1.
Housing.
Local government organization and administration.
Town and country planning.
Water supply, sewerage and sewage disposal.

Health and Social Security, Department of
(i) *Health* – Alexander Fleming House, Elephant and Castle, London, SE1.
Hospital and specialist services.
General medical and dental services, pharmaceutical services, supplementary ophthalmic services.
Health and welfare services provided by local authorities.
Children in care of local authorities and voluntary organizations.
Welfare foods and food hygiene.
Medical aspects of environmental services (water supplies, cleansing, sewerage, etc.).
Scotland: *Scottish Home and Health Department*, St Andrew's House, Edinburgh 1.
Wales: *Welsh Board of Health*, Cathays Park, Cardiff.
(ii) *Social Security* – 10 John Adam Street, London, WC2.
Family allowances, industrial injuries, national insurance, family income supplement and war pensions schemes.
(iii) *Supplementary Benefits Commission* – New Court, Carey Street, London, WC1.
Supplementary benefits and allowances, including higher rate scheme for the blind (there are no longer higher rates for the tuberculous).
Reception centres for persons without a settled way of life.
Re-establishment centres.
Investigation of resources for some applicants for legal aid.

Home Nursing

Home Office
Whitehall, London, SW1.
Treatment of offenders.
Prisons and borstals.
Police and probation services.
Immigrants and aliens.

Scottish Office
Dover House, Whitehall, London, SW1.
St Andrew's House, Edinburgh 1.

Welsh Office
Gwydyr House, Whitehall, London, SW1.
Cathays Park, Cardiff.

Northern Ireland
Development, Ministry of
Stormont, Belfast.
Housing.
Planning.
Local Government.

Home Affairs, Ministry of
Stormont, Belfast 4.
Law and justice.
Children in care (until 1974).

Health and Social Services, Ministry of
Dundonald House, Upper Newtownards Road, Belfast.
Hospital, health and welfare services.
Social security services.
Employment services.

Appendix

Food	Quantity	Calories
Almonds	1 oz	170
Anchovies	1 oz	50
Apple – 1 raw, approx. 2–2½ inches	4 oz	52
Apple – baked without sugar	4 oz	44
Apple – stewed without sugar	4 oz	36
Apricots – fresh	1 oz	8
Apricots – canned in syrup	1 oz	30
Apricots – dried, raw	1 oz	52
Asparagus – boiled	1 oz	5
Avocado	1 oz	25
Bacon – average rasher raw	1 oz	115
Bacon – average rasher fried (back)	1 oz	169
Bacon – average rasher fried (collar)	1 oz	124
Bacon – average rasher fried (gammon)	1 oz	126
Bacon – average rasher fried (streaky)	1 oz	149
Banana – one large	5 oz	110
Beans – green or french, boiled	1 oz	2
Beans – haricot, boiled	1 oz	25
Beans – canned, baked	1 oz	26
Beef – consomme	1 oz	approx. 4
Beef – corned	1 oz	66
Beef – roast topside, lean only	1 oz	71
Beef – roast topside, lean and fat	1 oz	91
Beef – roast sirloin, lean only	1 oz	64
Beef – roast sirloin, lean and fat	1 oz	109
Beef – boiled silverside	1 oz	86
Beef steak – raw	1 oz	50
Beef steak – fried	1 oz	78
Beef steak – grilled	1 oz	86
Beef steak – stewed	1 oz	58
Beer – Bitter	1 oz	90
Beer – Light Ale (bottled)	1 oz	90
Beer – Extra Stout	1 oz	110

Food	Quantity	Calories
Beetroot – boiled or canned	1 oz	13
Biscuits – water	1 oz	126
Biscuits – digestive, etc. (to serve with cheese)	1 oz	137
Biscuits – salted	1 oz	143
Biscuits – sweet	1 oz	158
Blackberries – raw	1 oz	8
Blackberries – sweetened, canned	1 oz	24
Blackcurrants – raw	1 oz	8
Blackcurrants – canned, sweetened	1 oz	21
Brains	1 oz	41·8
Brazil nuts	1 oz	183
Bread – white, brown	1 oz	69
Bread – rye	1 oz	68
Bread – wholemeal	1 oz	65
Bread – crispbread	1 oz	98
Bread – starch reduced (Procea)	1 oz	118–128
Bread – starch reduced rolls (Energen)	1 oz	111
Broccoli – boiled	1 oz	4
Brussels sprouts – boiled	1 oz	5
Butter	1 oz	226
Buttermilk	1 oz	10
Cabbage – raw	1 oz	7
Cabbage – boiled	1 oz	3
Cake – fruit (Dundee type)	1 oz	110
Cake – plain, sweet	1 oz	80
Cake – sponge	1 oz	87
Carrots – raw	1 oz	6
Carrots – boiled	1 oz	6
Cauliflower – cooked	1 oz	3
Celery – raw	1 oz	3
Cereals – cornflakes	1 oz	104
Cereals – oatmeal or porridge oats	1 oz	115
Cereals – starch reduced flakes	1 oz	114
Cereals – All Bran	1 oz	88
Cereals – Rice Crispies	1 oz	100
Cereals – Puffed Wheat	1 oz	102
Cereals – Weetabix	1 oz	100
Cheese – Camembert	1 oz	88
Cheese – Cheddar	1 oz	120

Food	Quantity	Calories
Cheese – Cottage	1 oz	32
Cheese – Gruyère	1 oz	132
Cheese – Processed	1 oz	106
Cheese – Parmesan	1 oz	118
Cheese – Spread	1 oz	82
Cheese – Stilton	1 oz	135
Cherries – fresh	1 oz	11
Cherries – canned, sweetened	1 oz	30
Chicken – grilled (edible meat)	1 oz	54
Chicken – roast, no fat or skin	1 oz	54
Chicken – stewed or boiled, no sauce	1 oz	58
Chives	for flavour	trace
Chocolate – plain	1 oz	155
Chocolate – milk	1 oz	167
Chocolate eclair (varies according to recipe)	1 oz	150–200
Chocolate sauce (varies according to recipe)	1 oz	90–150
Chop suey – canned	1 oz	120
Cocoa Powder (containing milk)	1 oz	128
Cod – steamed or poached	1 oz	23
Cod – fried (as purchased)	1 oz	58
Coffee – black	1 oz	1
Coffee – white (add amount of milk or cream)	1 oz	1
Consommé	1 oz	4
Corn on the Cob	1 ear	84
Cornflakes – see cereals		
Crab (weighed without shell)	1 oz	36
Cream – double	1 oz	131
Cream – single	1 oz	62
Cucumber	1 oz	3
Currants – dried	1 oz	76
Custard	1 oz	22
Dates – weighed with stones	1 oz	61
Duck – roast	1 oz	89
Egg – raw (standard)	2 oz	92
Egg – yolk (standard)	1 oz	99
Egg – white (standard)	1 oz	11
Fish	See under types	

Food	*Quantity*	*Calories*
Fruit jelly (packet)	1 oz	73
Grapefruit	1 oz	3
Grapefruit juice, sweetened	1 oz	19·5
Grapefruit juice, unsweetened	1 oz	7
Grapes – white	1 oz	17
Grapes – black	1 oz	14
Haddock – steamed or poached	1 oz	28
Haddock – fried	1 oz	50
Haddock – smoked	1 oz	28
Halibut – steamed or poached	1 oz	37
Ham – boiled, lean	1 oz	62
Ham – boiled, lean and fat	1 oz	123
Herring – fried	1 oz	67
Herring – soused	1 oz	54
Honey	1 oz	82
Horlicks	1 oz	113
Ice cream	1 oz	56
Jam or jelly and marmalade	1 oz	74
Jams – sugarless	1 oz	73
Kidney – ox, stewed	1 oz	45
Kidney, ox, fried	1 oz	57
Kippers – baked with bones and skin	1 oz	31
Lamb – chop, grilled, lean and fat	1 oz	142
Lamb – leg, roasted or stewed, lean	1 oz	83
Leeks – boiled	1 oz	7
Lemon – whole	1 oz	4
Lemon – juice, unsweetened	1 oz	2
Lentils – weighed after boiling	1 oz	27
Lettuce	1 oz	3
Liver – grilled	1 oz	41
Liver – fried	1 oz	74
Lobster – weighed without shell	1 oz	34
Luncheon meat	1 oz	95
Macaroni – boiled (and spaghetti)	1 oz	32
Marrow (courgettes, etc.) – boiled	1 oz	2
Mayonnaise	1 oz	150
Melon (average slice is 4 oz)	1 oz	7
Milk – whole	1 oz	19
Milk – skimmed	1 oz	10
Milk – evaporated	1 oz	45

Food	*Quantity*	*Calories*
Milk – condensed, full cream sweetened	1 oz	100
Mint jelly		Varies
Mint sauce, sweetened, sugar substitute	1 tblesp.	1
Mushrooms – raw or boiled	1 oz	2
Mushrooms – fried	1 oz	62
Mussels – weighed with shells, boiled	1 oz	7
Mustard	1 oz	trace
Mutton – leg, stewed	1 oz	74
Mutton – scrag end neck, stewed	1 oz	92
Noodles and other pasta	1 oz	109
Oil	1 oz	200–261
Olives – green and black (5 approx.)	1 oz	35–50
Onion – raw	1 oz	7
Onion – boiled	1 oz	4
Onion – fried	1 oz	101
Orange – medium approx. 5 oz	1 whole	40–50
Orange – unsweetened juice	1 oz	11
Orange – sweetened		Varies
Ovaltine and malted milk	1 oz	109
Pancakes – 4 inches	1 whole	60
Parsley	1 oz	6
Parsnips – boiled	1 oz	16
Peach – fresh, 1 approx.	5 oz	55
Peach – sweetened, canned	1 oz	25
Peanut butter	1 oz	118
Peanuts	1 oz	171
Pear – medium fresh	5 oz	40–50
Pear – canned in syrup	1 oz	22
Peas – fresh or canned, garden	1 oz	18
Peas – canned, processed	1 oz	24
Peas – dried	1 oz	78
Pepper	—	—
Peppers – capsicum	1 oz	10
Pickles – vinegar	1 oz	approx. 15
Pickles – mustard	1 oz	approx. 27
Pickles – sweet or chutney		Varies
Pineapple – fresh	1 oz	13
Pineapple – canned in syrup	1 oz	22

Food	Quantity	Calories
Pineapple – juice, canned, sweetened	1 oz	15
Plaice – steamed	1 oz	26
Plaice – fried	1 oz	66
Plums – fresh	1 oz	11
Plums – stewed without sugar	1 oz	6
Pork – roast loin, lean and fat	1 oz	129
Pork – roast loin, very lean	1 oz	90
Pork – chops, grilled, lean and fat	1 oz	155
Pork – chops, grilled, lean only	1 oz	92
Porridge	1 oz	115
Port – Red	1 oz	43
Potatoes – boiled	1 oz	23
Potatoes – baked in skins	1 oz	30
Potatoes – roast	1 oz	35
Potatoes – chips	1 oz	68
Potatoes – crisps	1 oz	159
Prawns – fresh peeled, frozen or canned	1 oz	30
Prunes – raw with stones	1 oz	38
Prunes – stewed without sugar, with stones	1 oz	19
Rabbit – stewed	1 oz	51
Radishes	1 oz	4
Raisins	1 oz	70
Raspberries – raw	1 oz	7
Raspberries – frozen or canned with sugar	1 oz	25
Rhubarb – cooked with sugar substitute	1 oz	1
Rice – boiled	1 oz	35
Rolls (see bread also)	1 medium	approx. 115
Rolls	1 large	approx. 155
Salad Cream	1 oz	111
Salami	1 oz	90
Salmon – fresh, poached or steamed	1 oz	57
Salmon – canned	1 oz	39
Salt	—	—
Sardines – canned, drained	1 oz	84
Sausages – pork, fried	1 oz	93
Sausages – beef, fried	1 oz	81

Food	Quantity	Calories
Scallops – poached	1 oz	30
Sherry – Dry	1 oz	33
Sherry – Sweet	1 oz	38
Shrimps – fresh peeled, frozen or canned	1 oz	32
Sole – steamed	1 oz	24
Sole – fried	1 oz	78
Soup – thick	1 oz	Varies 80 upwards
Soy sauce	1 oz	10
Spinach – boiled	1 oz	7
Spirits – 70% proof	1 oz	63
Squash – lemon and orange	1 oz	39
Squash – Ribena	1 oz	65
Strawberries – fresh	1 oz	7
Strawberries – canned or frozen with sugar	1 oz	24
Suet	1 oz	262
Sugar – all kinds	1 oz	112
Sugar substitute	1 oz	—
Swede – boiled	1 oz	5
Sweetmeats	1 oz	approx. 120
Syrup – golden	1 oz	84
Tangerine	1 oz	10
Tea	1 oz	—
Tomato – raw	1 oz	4
Tomato – fried	1 oz	20
Tomato – juice	1 oz	6
Tomato – ketchup	1 oz	28
Tongue	1 oz	88
Treacle – Black	1 oz	73
Tripe – cooked without milk	1 oz	29
Trout – steamed	1 oz	38
Tuna fish – canned	1 oz	40
Turkey – roast	1 oz	56
Turnip – boiled	1 oz	3
Veal – lean roast fillet	1 oz	66
Veal – grilled cutlet no bone	1 oz	60
Veal – fried cutlet no bone	1 oz	61
Vinegar	1 oz	1

Appendix

Food	Quantity	Calories
Walnuts	1 oz	156
Watercress	1 oz	4
Water ice (sorbet)	1 oz	30
White sauce	1 oz	41
Whiting – steamed	1 oz	26
Whiting – fried	1 oz	55
Wines – Dry	1 oz	21
Wines – Sweet	1 oz	26
Yoghurt (low fat) natural	1 oz	15
Yoghurt (low fat) fruit	1 oz	30
Yoghurt (low fat) hazel nut	1 oz	37

Index

Compiled by Jo Cape

Index

Index

Phenylketonuria, 201, 207–8
Physical disability, care of person with, 211–36
Piles, 174–5
Pillows, 23
Play, 99–100, 160, 209–10
Poisoning, 243–5, 299–302
Poliomyelitis, 135–6, 211
  vaccine, 129, 130
Polypus, 120
Post mortem, 191
Poultices, 76
Pressure sores, 46–9
Prostate gland, post-operative care, 174
Psychoses, 196–200
  puerpal, 199–200
  senile, 198
Pulmonary valve stenosis, 172
Pulse rate, 38

Radiotherapy, 155–6
Rash, 33
Reading aids, 228
Regional Health Authority, 310
Respiration rate, 38–9
Resuscitation, 248–53
Rhesus testing, 200
Ribs, fracture, 289–91
Ringworm, 148
Rubella see German measles
Rupture, 302–3

Scabies, 143
Scarlet fever, 134
Schizophrenia, 176–7
  autism, 208–9
Shaving a patient, 45
Sheets, 23, 25
Shingles, 140–1
Shock, 305–7
Sickroom, 11–17, 183–4
Skin, 33, 137–43
  foreign body in, 280
Sleep, baby, 97
  children, 100–1
  insomnia, 181–2
  after stroke, 152
Slipped disc, 154
Smallpox, vaccination, 128–9, 130
Smoking, heart attack, 152
Social services, 312
Spastic, 203, 211
Spina bifida, 175–6
Spinal injuries, 287–9
Splints, 285
Sputum, observation, 39
Steroids, 56
Stomach, foreign body in, 280
Stools, babies, 97–8
  observation, 39
Strain, muscular, 304

Sunburn, 304–5
Street accidents, 245–6
Strokes, 149, 150, 252–3, 305
Suicide, 301
Surgery, care after, 170–6
Syphilis, 120–1

Tables for disabled, 229
Tapeworm, 115
Teeth, care of, 43–4
Telephone aids, 229
Temperature, taking, 35–7
Testes, undescended, 112–13
Tetanus, 135
  vaccination, 129
Thermometer, 35
Threadworms, 115
Throat, foreign body in, see Choking
Thrombosis, cerebral, 144
  coronary, 144
Thrush, 120, 141
Thumb-sucking, 113
Toilet, 41–53, 178–9, 216, 224
Tonsilitis, 136
  tonsilectomy, 176–7
Tuberculosis, BCG, 129
Typhoid and paratyphoid fevers, 134–5

Ulcers, peptic, diet for, 57
Urine, observation, 39
  urinals, 51–3

Vaccination, 128–9
Vagina, discharges, 119–20
  warts, 120
Varicose veins, piles, 174
Venereal diseases, 120–1
Ventilation, sick room, 13
Ventricular sepial defect, 172–3
Vitamins, 55, 64–5
Voluntary services, 314; addresses, 315–52
Vomit, 179; in infants, 85
  observations, 39
  peptic ulcers, 153

Warts, 139
Water retention see Oedema
Weight, gaining diet, 62–3
  reducing diet, 60–1
Wheelchairs, 226–7
Whooping cough, 131–2
  immunity, 128
  vaccination, 129
Wind, 88
Winding, 307
Worms, 115
Writing aids, 228–9

X-ray treatment, 155

Yeast infections, 141

368